M000280655

Healthy by *Design*

Healthy Eating, God's Way

Weight Loss Devotional and Challenge

Calm your Cravings, Overcome
Obsessing, Hone Healthy Habits, and
Build Biblical Boundaries.

Cathy Morenzie

Guiding Light Publishing

Published: June 2021

ISBN: (print) 978-1-990078-01-9
(digital) 978-1-990078-02-6

Published by Guiding Light Publishing
46 Bell St, Barrie, ON, Canada, L4N 0H9

Note: The information in this book is for educational purposes only and is not recommended as a means of diagnosing or treating illness. All situations concerning physical or mental health should be supervised by a health professional knowledgeable in treating that particular condition. Neither the author nor anyone affiliated with Healthy by Design dispenses medical advice, nor do they prescribe any remedies or assume any responsibility for anyone who chooses to treat themselves.

Cover and author photo by: martinbrownphotography.com

Interior Design by: Davor Dramikanin

Table of Contents

Preface

Welcome, my friend! I'm thrilled that you're here to discover just what *'Healthy Eating, God's Way'* means. Let me put your mind at ease, it has nothing to do with eating locusts and wild honey like John the Baptist, nor will you have to sacrifice all of your favourite foods.

Healthy Eating, God's Way might look like this for you... Imagine waking up tomorrow, no alarm, no need to hit the snooze button, you're feeling energized, refreshed, and can't wait to start the day. You grab a glass of water with some lemon in it and spend some sweet time in praise and worship. During your prayer time, you commit your day to the Lord. You ask Him to guide all of your eating choices and thank Him for giving you a spirit of self-control and discipline. You then cue up one of your favourite *Get Active, God's Way* workouts to kick start your day then head to the kitchen. What will you eat today? You check in with your body and it's telling you that you're not very hungry and have a cup of tea as you think about what you're going to eat for lunch and dinner. Your friend calls and invites you out to lunch, but you gracefully decline because you know that you always overeat when you go out with her. Thankfully, you've already planned out your meals for the week so you see that for lunch you'll be feasting on a delicious salad with chicken breast, and for dinner you'll be enjoying a scrumptious bowl of butternut squash soup. You eat your meals slowly, enjoying every bite and giving God thanks for all that was involved to get these meals to your table. You finish your last meal at 7:00 pm and think about if you'll spend your evening completing one of your special projects or calling a couple of friends for fellowship time. You do both. You feel so satisfied and content with your day that snacking does not even cross your mind. So you spend some time journaling, giving God thanks for the day, and go to sleep soundly.

Sound like a fairy tale?

What if I told you that this could be you within the next month?

Sure, it might seem nothing like your life right now, but once you read *Healthy Eating, God's Way*, your eyes will be opened to what's possible.

Right now, you may be so stuck in your habits and routines that you can't imagine ever changing. Or maybe you've tried so many times that you don't believe that anything will work.

It's not your fault!

You've been led to believe that if only you were eating the right foods and doing the right things, then... Like winning the lottery, if only you could crack the code on the right combination of foods, timing, ratios, and quantities then you'd hit that jackpot, but it's all a myth. You've been looking for a secret formula that simply does not exist!

And that's why this book is so important. I wrote *Healthy Eating, God's Way* in response to the ago old question: "What should I eat?" Here's the thing... You're asking the wrong question! Asking what you should eat assumes that when you get the answer, you'll learn what to eat, eat it, and reap all the rewards. Right? Except knowledge is not the problem, it's the application of what you know that's the real problem. If you're honest with yourself, you already know what to eat but you still don't do it.

Here's why: Unless you've been living off the grid for most of your life, I'm pretty sure you know what to eat—vegetables, fruits, nuts, seeds, whole grains, to avoid processed foods and other foods with little or no nutritional value. It's that simple, but what people really want to know are questions like:

Should I be eating paleo or keto?

Should I be intermittent fasting and if so, what should my window be?

What are the best low carbohydrate foods to eat?

Is Stevia ok to use instead of sugar?

Are diet sodas okay?

What will help to reduce my sugar cravings?

Maybe you've asked yourself these questions. Or maybe you have a list of other perplexing health questions.

Healthy Eating, God's Way will give you the answers to the right questions. Questions that will simplify your health and weight loss journey so that you don't waste your life trying to find answers to questions that only keep you spinning your wheels, overwhelmed and ever more confused. *Healthy Eating, God's Way* will take you back to simplicity by giving you biblical truths that will give you the framework to answer the unending questions that keep coming up in the trillion-dollar health and weight loss industry. Those types of questions will never stop, because every time we think we've finally figured it out the industry will come up with the next revolutionary diet.

A better question to ask instead of 'what should I eat,' is this: **"Why aren't you?"**

Why aren't you eating the foods that you know are nutritious?

Why aren't you able to resist all the tempting snacks and junk foods?

Why aren't you putting your fork down when you're already full?

Why aren't you eating within the boundaries you set for yourself?

When you take the time to answer those questions, that's when you will have a real breakthrough in your eating habits. When you confront the root of your emotional eating, cravings, and lack of what you think is self-control head on, that's when you will WANT to eat the foods that God designed to nourish your body. That's when paleo, keto, Whole30, or Atkins won't matter so much.

Listen, there's nothing wrong with any of these plans. In fact, they all work...if you work them, and that's where the breakdown will happen every time.

Healthy Eating, God's Way will take you back to simple eating. No good foods or bad foods, no points or calorie counting, and no starvation. When you understand and come into alignment with God's plan for your health, you don't have to stress about whether you're following all the rules of your program. Unlike the Pharisees who were always trying to over-complicate things and turn everything into a bunch of rules that they could never stick to, *Healthy Eating, God's Way* will help you break free from all of that confusion by getting back to God's essential truths.

By the end of this book you will gain an entirely new perspective on healthy eating—one that you may have never imagined was possible for you.

You will shift your focus from seeing healthy eating as a boring, tedious, and next to impossible goal to a simple, fun habit that energizes and revitalizes you. It will help you to find freedom from emotional eating and see food as medicine, as nourishment, and as a source of pleasure without feelings of guilt or shame. You'll look forward to your next meal!

As you go through this book, I'm also offering you many special bonus tools and templates to support you on this journey, such as:

- Weekly Meal Plan Template
- Healthy Eating Checklist
- Printable Healthy Eating Journal

Also, as an extra bonus you can also immediately download my '3 Steps to Overcoming Emotional Eating' guide to help you get fast-tracked right away. Use this repeatable three-step approach to reverse impulsive eating habits and turn your needs over to God instead. It's a quick read, so be sure to review this before starting the devotional part of this book.

One more thing... be sure to stay in touch with me so you can maintain your momentum as you read through this book.

healthyeatinggodswaybonus.com

Introduction

I wrote my first book, *Weight Loss, God's Way*, over 12 years ago, to help me with my own personal challenges with my own weight—although to look at me, you would never believe that this has been a lifelong battle. I knew that this was an idol in my life that took up too much mental energy and space in my head. I thought about food all day long, and deep down inside I knew that if I ever had to make the choice between God and my favourite food I'm not sure which one I'd choose. That scared me beyond belief.

When you're 300 or 400 pounds, it's easy to say, "I need help" and people will believe you, but when you're a personal fitness trainer who teaches others to lose weight, and who looks the part, then you're just an obsessive narcissist and a perfectionist who wants to have the perfect body. When I looked in the mirror, I did not see what others saw. I was only focused on the flaws and the cellulite around my hips and bum coupled with the taunts of the other children from the school yard still reverberated in my head from my childhood; "Big-batty-Cathy," they would laugh and tease. 'Batty' was the word for bum in many of the Caribbean Islands.

Since I was so insecure, broken, prideful, gluttonous and ashamed, it was so much easier to live the lie that everyone wanted to believe about me than to face the truth. So that's what I did for most of my adult life as I outwardly played the part of 'fitness guru', but inwardly I suffered in silence.

Anyone I attempted to talk to about it seemed to roll their eyes at me. "What do you have to worry about? You have the perfect body," they would say dismissively. Since no one else knew my struggles because on the outside I looked to be the picture of health, I stopped sharing my pain. I would binge eat and then use Ex Lax or jump on the cabbage soup diet, Master Cleanse, or whatever the quick trending weight loss diet was for a few days to get my weight back down. This went on from my teens well into my 40s. I used to love our annual church fast in February because that was a way to get my weight down, and it gave me a legitimate reason. But as soon as March hit, I'd start obsessing about food again.

So I stopped talking about it and began to take everything I had learned in the health and fitness industry and tried to understand it all from a biblical perspective; goal-setting, procrastinating, self-control, excuse-making. I studied God's Word, taking all the head knowledge I had learned in university and my post-grad studies and set out on the journey to end this cycle of guilt and shame. My goal—to surrender this mind obsessed about food, health, and weight to God.

As selfish as it sounds, I wrote *Weight Loss, God's Way* to help myself. I wrote about all of the areas that I had been struggling with and then I read what the bible had to say on each of the topics. I studied bible characters who struggled with similar issues, although they were not directly related to health or weight.

I was afraid that people would think that I was trying to use the bible for something as trite as weight loss. I thought that people would not make the connection between their faith and their weight and they would not be open to the idea of inviting God into this intimate area of their lives. Turns out I was wrong about what people thought. My story hit a chord with women from all over the world, and men too. I was not alone in my struggles, but I did not know this for some years after writing *Weight Loss, God's Way* because I parked it on the shelf—for years!

But God always has a plan despite our fears and false beliefs. He sent my husband who happened to be 'dabbling' in self-publishing. What are the odds? LOL. He pulled my dusty book off the shelf and published it on Amazon. The response from women all over the world was remarkable. As others read *Weight Loss, God's Way* they were shocked that they'd never even thought of inviting God into their weight releasing journey, but they're so glad they did. As they turned their weight struggles over to God, He worked in their lives to transform their health in ways that they never thought they would ever experience.

It's now been 13 years since I wrote the first edition of *Weight Loss, God's Way*, and I'm a lot older and wiser. I've submitted my weight releasing journey to God and it's made all the difference. Many of the habits that I've struggled to maintain most of my adult life are now routine, with only small blips in my routine mostly at Christmas and holidays. But there's still one area that I've yet to experience a breakthrough in and that's the area of food.

And that's why I set out to write this devotional. To invite women to join me once again on my journey towards submitting this stronghold to God in this devotional, *Healthy Eating, God's Way*.

Healthy eating is just one of the many aspects of managing a healthy weight, and for most of us it's the biggest to overcome. It's definitely the case for me. 'Experts' say that managing your weight is 75% what you eat and 25% exercise. Despite those statistics, I believe that God is 100% in control and that's why I refuse to give up or give in. As I write this in my 50s, I believe that at any age in our life we can take control of what we eat. It's never too late, you're never too young or too old to take control of the foods you eat. But not the way you've been going about it. It's time to flip the paradigm of healthy eating for weight loss on its head. So that's exactly what I will do as I share my daily inspirations, meditations, and prescriptions with you.

Like *Weight Loss, God's Way* and my other books, I will not approach *Healthy Eating, God's Way* as a how-to book to eat healthfully and manage my weight, but rather as a guide that I can refer to each time I need to remember why it's important to choose salads over sweets and water or wine. *Healthy Eating, God's Way* is my North-star, my guiding light that keeps me grounded in God's truth so that I can always find my way back when I veer off course.

So I invite you to follow me as I follow Christ in this journey towards nourishing my temple.

I'm writing this devotional to remind myself and you that this is an emotional battle which, like all emotional battles, requires spiritual solutions.

So I encourage you as I encourage myself to know that you can be free from the hold that food has on you right now. It does not require your belief right now, it does not require you to have a big vision. All that's required is that you will commit to get into God's Word and study for yourself how He wants to free you from anything and everything that robs you of your peace, joy, and freedom.

What to Expect as you Read this Book

I'm an avid reader.

This allows me to appreciate books from both vantage points. As a reader, I appreciate knowing ahead of time what I can expect so that I can manage my expectations and pace myself for what is to come.

Expect Resistance

I'll be the first to admit that I've stopped reading books when the material was 'hard', or it started ruffling my feathers. I know it's good for me, but my flesh was not prepared to receive it. So now you're sufficiently forewarned. You may experience resistance as you read this book. Resistance is push-back from yourself that you will feel. It is part of the process of growth and change. Don't be surprised when it comes. Some resistance is God perfecting us, and some is the enemy keeping us from our victory. Discern which is which, and exercise the power of prayer accordingly.

Yes, you may want to quit. Yes, the enemy will try to convince you that you can't do it. Know that victory is waiting on the other side.

"Consider it pure joy, my brothers and sisters, whenever you face trials of many kinds because you know that the testing of your faith produces perseverance. Let perseverance finish its work so that you may be mature and complete, not lacking anything." ~James 1:2-4

Expect to Work

You will get out of this book exactly what you put in. If you don't do the work, then you cannot expect to see a change.

"Whatever you do, work at it with all your heart, as working for the Lord, not for men, since you know that you will receive an inheritance from the Lord as a reward. It is the Lord Christ you are serving." ~ Col. 3:23-25

Expect Renewed Joy and Hope in the Lord

Something beautiful begins to happen when you spend more time with the Lord. He will minister to your heart and soul. Expect that your relationship with the Lord will be strengthened as a result of this journey.

Expect to Feel Fear

Fear is at the root of most of the things that stop us in life.

As you read this book, all kinds of fears may come out of the woodwork. Fear of injury, fear of failure, fear of commitment. Just be aware of them and know that, in due season, they will be dealt with. Resist the urge to try to confront too many fears at once. Just know that it exists, and resist the urge to run and hide when you experience it.

Expect Changes in your Patterns

Are you always doing things at the last minute, then wondering why things don't work out for you?

Maybe you do not take the time to plan what you will eat. There will be habits that you notice that will get in the way of your success—journal them and turn them over to the Lord. You can't change everything at once, but you should make note of it for future reference.

How to Read this Book

First. Accountability!

Enlist a trusted friend to study this devotional with you. Accountability is always an important key to any journey, because we are always more successful together than alone. An accountability partner will challenge you, support you, and allow you to see blind spots that you may not otherwise see. Who can you think who also needs support to eat healthier? Invite them to read this book with you.

I suggest you read through the 28 days of the devotional, one day at a time. The goal is to allow God to change you from the inside out. This is a process, and it takes time. If you rush through it, you will miss the gold that God has for you in the pages of this book.

Most of the 28 days contain seven sections: scripture reflection, devotion, action, reflect, pray, my prayer, and additional scriptures.

Below are some instructions on how to use each of these sections. Don't feel like you need to do all of them each day.

Scripture Reflection:

> *"Oh, how I love your law! I meditate on it all day long."*
> *~Psalm 119:97*

Study the daily scripture as you go about your day.

Write it down, ask the Holy Spirit to bring it to your remembrance when appropriate. Put it on your fridge or on the dashboard of your car—anywhere you will be able to refer to it a few times a day. It's the Word of God that has the power to change us to meditate on His word.

Devotion:

"So we have come to know and to believe the love that God has for us. God is love, and whoever abides in love abides in God, and God abides in him."
(1 John 4:16)

The devotion introduces the main topic in both a practical and spiritual context. Read it to understand how the Holy Spirit is leading and guiding you. Each devotion is designed to bring you back to the overarching truth, that God is calling you to rethink healthy eating from His perspective, and He promises to be with you on your journey.

Action:

It's far too easy to just read something, nod our head in agreement, but never take action. This section is designed to get you into action right away. Each day you will take one small step towards healthier eating, God's way. Remember it's just one day, so don't worry about whether you will be able to maintain it. Take small daily steps in faith and leave the rest to God.

Reflect:

Life can get so busy. Even our devotion time can become something else on our to-do list. Taking time to reflect allows us to slow down and think about how the daily topics affect you and your relationship with God. The daily reflection will give you a better understanding of yourself in light of the Word of God. Read the questions at the start of the day and reflect on them throughout the day.

Pray:

Enjoy the daily guided prayer. Sometimes it can be difficult to articulate what's in your heart, so I've provided you with guided prayers that you can make your own to cry out to God.

Each prayer is a beautiful summary of the daily scripture and devotion.

My Prayer:

In addition to the guided prayer, I encourage you to take some time and journal your personal prayers to God, sharing your heart with Him. Pour your heart out to God. Speak His Word back to Him; confess, declare, supplicate, and cry out to Him in prayer. James 5:16 teaches us that the prayer of a righteous person is powerful and effective.

Additional Scriptures:

I've included some additional scriptures at the end of each day if you want to delve deeper into the topic. God's Word is so rich and powerful. The more you study His Word the greater your insight will become.

Ready? Let's go!

DEVOTIONAL

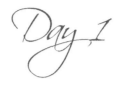

Food as a Gift from God

Scripture Reflection

"And people should eat and drink and enjoy the fruits of their labor, for these are gifts from God." ~ *Ecclesiastes 3:13*

Overview

My husband often wishes that he could just take a pill everyday that fills his belly so he does not have to think about food. To him, food is an annoyance and an inconvenience that interrupts his day. I'm the exact opposite...from the moment I wake up, I think about food. It's one of the highlights of my day and, unlike my hubby, I think that much of my life is centered around it. Because it's that important for me, it's important that it's nutritious.

If you're anything like me, food fills your thoughts, conversations, time, and energy. Whether it's planning, tracking, shopping, preparing, or eating, the goal is to eat nutritious, nourishing foods that leave me feeling satisfied and content.

Despite how much attention we give food, we are no wiser about how to stop ourselves from the lure of un-nutritious foods, or how we're to eat to maintain a healthy weight once we have achieved it.

It's enough for us to want to surrender with the white flag and say, "Pass the Häagen-Dazs!"

We're so busy trying to figure out calories, points, and the latest low-carb foods that it allows the enemy to have a field day with us. He's won again by keeping us distracted and focusing on minutiae that was never meant to take up so much of our time.

We've made food a mystery to be solved, a puzzle to be pieced together, and a vault to be entered into with a magical combination. But it's so much more than any of these approaches. Food is a gift from God (Ecc. 3:13) and the sooner we can see it from this perspective, the sooner we will be free from the bondage of food and its minions of guilt, shame, and bewilderment.

So just how do you have a conversation about healthy eating without making food the enemy? That's what we're about to explore.

This devotional will give a biblical approach to healthy eating—especially as it relates to weight release. More importantly, it will give you the freedom to enjoy nutritious food without turning it into a production, feeling like you need a degree in food science to figure it all out. You will learn that you can eat in a way that honors God as you learn to honor your temple. Though the Bible doesn't specifically talk about eating for weight release, there are numerous passages that talk about food, dietary practices, gluttony, discipline, self-control, eating clean food, cooking food and specific foods—all essential topics related to healthy eating.

Someone once wisely said that "there is only one way to eat an elephant: a bite at a time." This means that everything in life that seems overwhelming and even impossible can be accomplished gradually by taking it one step at a time or one bit at a time. That's exactly how you will approach this devotional and challenge. One day at a time, one small challenge at a time. Each day will introduce you to one small principle that you will practice for that day. Surely you can do anything for just one day, right?

Get ready to challenge yourself each day. Get ready to discover how to eat healthfully and how to make choices that honor God with your body! Know that this important decision about what is "healthy" has to do with more than just the nutrition facts label! You will discover how your health impacts your body, soul, AND spirit.

In this devotional you will:

- Develop an appreciation of God's gift of food
- Practice a daily healthy eating challenge
- Understand what you're really craving
- Develop a biblical model for healthy weight release
- Study what God's Word says about food and healthy eating
- Learn how to put and keep food in its proper place in your life
- Practice healthy eating habits

Action

Just for today... Start the process by establishing a starting point. Sign up for MyFitnessPal, or another tracking tool. Watch this training video to learn how:

weightlossgodsway.com/myfitnesspal

Reflect

1. What's your biggest challenge with healthy eating? Emotional eating? Portion control? Late-night eating?

_____

_____

_____

_____

_____

Prayer

"Lord, I thank You that You and You alone will satisfy me. Despite my attempts to find the right foods to end these cravings, I know that true satisfaction can only come from You. So as I embark on this time of searching for the right foods and right diets, remind me that it's not about what I eat that will make me feel whole, but what You can and will do in my life when I lay down all of my idols and everything that keeps me from having fellowship with You. As I discover new insights in this devotional, remind me that information without revelation from You will not transform me, so I continue to press into You. I feed on Your Word and move away from everything that keeps me from having sweet communion with You. It's Your Word that I'm really craving, and I purpose to stay full of it each and every day. In Your Holy Name, I pray. Amen!"

My Prayer

_____

_____

_____

_____

_____

_____

_____

_____

_____

_____

_____

_____

_____

_____

_____

_____

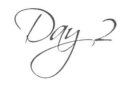

Search Me O God–Really!

Scripture Reflection

> *"Search me, O God, and know my heart. See if there is any*
> *offensive way in me, and lead me in the way everlasting."*
> *~Psalm 139:23-24*

Devotion

Here I go again. I'm about to embark upon yet another program to help me get my eating under control.

If you're of my generation, you'll remember the cartoon show *The Jetsons* where George Jetson is stuck on this perpetual treadmill, screaming to his wife, "Help, Jane! Stop this crazy thing!" That's how I feel about my relationship with food.

I've been here far too many times and know that I'm no match for my powerful cravings. They just seem to come out of nowhere. They remind me of how, like Esau (Genesis 25:29-34), I'll easily give up my birthright to satisfy my appetite, and so now on top of a scoop of guilt I've added an extra serving of shame. That'll teach me to overeat. But it doesn't.

I'm so tired of it! I'm tired of the guilt and shame. I'm tired of feeling like I'm always choosing food over God. And I'm tired of feeling like I'm always starting over. I know that when I call out to Him He will help me, but in truth, when those cravings come, I want the food more than I want God. Ugh. It pains me to even admit it. It's in this place of guilt that can no longer be ignored or pacified that I cry out to God for help and I know that He will answer me.

But before we start confessing and declaring "in Jesus' Name" to help us overcome our food addictions and strongholds, let's deal with the elephant in the room. Sometimes, this Christian thing does not work. If it always did, then why is our divorce rate as high as non-Christians and our rate of obesity even higher than non-Christians? What's up with that? How long will we hide our head in the sand as we say "praise the Lord and pass the biscuits."

If this is going to be another devotional that you're in a rush to get through so that you can do your "morning devotion-check," I'm going to warn you this ain't that kind of devotion. I'm coming hard this time because sugar-coating our disobedience in clichès and "Christianese" just ain't cutting it for me anymore. I want real change! I want change that goes beyond reading a devotional or book.

So let's start with a deep dive into the heart of the matter. Let's challenge ourselves to invite God in and ask Him to search our hearts. Yes, I know you've done it before, but have you really?

Henry Melvill, a renowned British priest in the Church of England, warns, "I call upon you to be cautious in using this prayer. It is easy to mock God, by asking Him to search you whilst you have made but little effort to search yourselves, and perhaps still less to act upon the result of the scrutiny."

Are you ready to truly pray this prayer, perhaps in a way like never before? If so, will you then take the time to listen to what He says as a result? Will you commit to then act upon it and allow Him to change you? Jesus stated, "Without me you can do nothing" (John 15:5). We must be part of the vine. When we're connected to Him, He will do the work of changing us because, as you've probably already noticed from your past attempts, you can't change yourself.

As you embark, don't just make this like every other devotional. Purpose in your heart that you will not make this another "feel good, nod your head in agreement with what you read, but not really change" kind of devotional. Don't just "try again" to get your eating under control. Search yourself and make sure that you are truly ready and willing to do what you hear the Lord telling you to do. If not, you'll end up just continuing to stay stuck. Like the man waiting at the pool for a miracle (John 5:6), it's time to answer the question: "Do you really want to get well?" "Do you really WANT to change this time? I don't know about you, sister, but I'm so tired of taking one step forward and two steps back.

Ready? Let's go!

Action

Just for today, read Psalms 139:23-34. Then read it again and ask God to search your heart and your mind to show you your anxious thoughts as they relate to your relationship with food. Then allow Him to show you one area in your relationship with food where you often break your boundaries. Choose only one. It could be:

- decreasing your salt content
- decreasing carbohydrate count
- tracking your food
- eliminating snacking
- eating more vegetables
- drinking more water

Whichever you choose, you will continue to focus on that 'Action Step' throughout the rest of this devotional study.

Reflect

1. Will you allow God to point out the sin in your life? Will you let Him truly show you the Way and lead you on the right path? He will lead us, but we must be willing to follow. Journal how He has been speaking to you in the past and journal how you have responded.

   _____

   _____

   _____

   _____

2. Repent and ask for forgiveness for not listening to His leading and guiding, or if you have listened then repent for not executing what He has shown you to do.

   _____

   _____

   _____

   _____

3. Do you really want to get well? Are you really ready to make the change?

   _____

   _____

   _____

   _____

Prayer

"Dear Lord, thank You for taking the time to explore my heart and show me the things in me that I'm unable to see with my own natural eyes. As You uncover evil ways in me, take them from me. I have so many blindspots that have been keeping me on a treadmill going nowhere, but I'm truly ready to surrender them to You. I don't want this book to be another thing where I just "give it a try." Let this be the defining moment where I commit to finally laying down what I keep picking up. No matter how entrenched my habits have become and no matter how far I've strayed from what healthy eating looks like, please deliver me from all of it. In Jesus' Name, Amen!"

My Prayer

_____

_____

_____

_____

_____

_____

_____

Additional Scriptures

"Who can discern his own errors? Cleanse me from my hidden faults." ~ Psalms 19:12

"Instead, we speak as those approved by God to be entrusted with the gospel, not in order to please men but God, who examines our hearts." ~ 1 Thes. 2:4

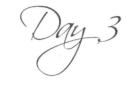

Getting Clear

Scripture Reflection

"Looking at him, Jesus showed love to him and said to him, 'One thing you lack: go and sell all you possess and give to the poor, and you will have treasure in heaven; and come, follow Me.' But he was deeply dismayed by these words, and he went away grieving; for he was one who owned much property." ~ Mark 10:21-22

Devotion

I pray that you're already feeling lighter and freer as you've fully surrendered your eating to God. Or maybe reality is kicking in and you're having a mild (or major) panic attack as you remember how this story has always ended in the past. Whatever you're feeling, it's all good. Accept that these feelings are normal and that you don't have to do anything more with them than feel them and remind yourself that, as we stay connected to Him, the Holy Spirit is now running the show, not your feelings. Isn't that a relief?

Today you're going to get clear on your goal and the actions required to achieve it. If you're anything like me, it's so easy to get caught up in the whirlwind of weight release so much so that you can no longer see the forest for the trees. For example, I've gotten so focused on tracking my food and maintaining my carb count that I forgot the reason I'm doing all of this in the first place. Tracking is not the goal, it's the means or the action step to get to the goal. In fact, achieving a healthy weight is not even the goal. The goal is living a healthy life so we can serve God more fully. Tracking my food and maintaining a healthy weight are the action steps that will allow the goal to be realized.

In Mark 10:21, the rich young ruler wanted to have something (eternal life), but he was not aware of the effort and sacrifice that it would take to obtain what he wanted. That's why it will be important for you to understand where you are now, where you want to get, and just what it will take to get there.

There's so much confusion in the health and fitness world about the goal and the action steps. We are of one of two mindsets:

1. We can get so caught up in the action steps, processes, and strategies that we lose sight of the ultimate goal. We become like the Pharisees who were caught up in rules and regulations that often missed the entire point of religion.

2. On the flip side, we can be like the rich young ruler with a sincere desire to want to achieve a goal—until we hear what it will really takes to have what we desire and recognize that we're not willing to do it.

Can you see yourself in any of these two scenarios? If so, take heart. You're in the right place. *Healthy eating, God's Way* requires a commitment to BOTH the action steps and the goal and that's what you will discover today.

So, let's get clear:

1. **Goal**- Your goal is the desired outcome you want to achieve. It can also be defined as a vision, which is a revelation from God. Your goal is not a place you're

trying to get to, but a return to who you already are in Christ. Our ultimate goal is holiness.

2. **Action Steps**– Action steps are the activities, habits, behaviors, and mindsets that you pursue on a daily basis to achieve your goal. They are not the goal in and of themselves, but the steps required to get there. Unless these action steps are leading you towards your goal, they're futile.

In the past, I've been so hyper-focused on tracking my food and maintaining my carb count that those practices became the goal. When you make the mistake and get so caught up with the action steps and forget the goal, you run the risk of missing the mark altogether and losing sight of the ultimate goal.

Action

Just for today, if it's not already obvious, spend some time in prayer and write out your health goal. Not your weight release goal. What do you want and why? Then pray and ask the Lord to show you a picture of what a healthy diet looks like for you. Either by creating a picture collage, or simply by writing it out as specifically as you can. You can flip through a magazine and cut out some photos or surf the Web to print out some images. Have fun!

Reflect

1. What are the long term implications or consequences of not achieving your health goal?

_____

_____

_____

_____

2. Review yesterday's lesson and recap what the Holy Spirit showed you about the healthy eating boundary that you continue to break. Ask yourself how this keeps you from achieving your ultimate health goal.

_____

_____

_____

_____

3. What adjustment is the Holy Spirit prompting you to make so that you can keep moving forward with your action step you chose on Day 2?

_____

_____

_____

_____

Prayer

"Dear Lord, I thank You for giving me clarity in the midst of the difficulties, trials, and temptations. I thank You that I only need to keep my eyes and my mind fixed on You and it is there that I will find focus, strength, clarity, and peace for this journey. Never let me get so caught up in the process that I miss You. I am getting healthier to bring You glory, not to check off a bunch of actions on my to-do list, or to lose weight. Losing weight is not the final goal; it's just one step on the journey that draws me closer to You as I remove all the blocks and hindrances. I thank You for helping me to take the necessary steps to be conformed into Your image and likeness. In Jesus' Name, Amen."

My Prayer

_____

_____

_____

_____

_____

_____

_____

_____

_____

_____

Additional Scriptures

And we all, who with unveiled faces contemplate the Lord's glory, are being transformed into his image with ever-increasing glory, which comes from the Lord, who is the Spirit. ~2 Corinthians 3:18

What goes into someone's mouth does not defile them, but what comes out of their mouth, that is what defiles them." ~Matthew 15:11

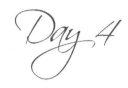

Measure It to Manage It

Scripture Reflection

"Wisdom is the principal thing; therefore get wisdom: and with all thy getting get understanding." ~Proverbs 4:7

Devotion

Like any journey you embark upon, it's important to have a roadmap. It will highlight the most efficient way to arrive at your destination in the quickest amount of time. A roadmap will keep you on track and keep you from wandering aimlessly. If you live in Toronto and want to go to New York, the roadmap will look very different from the map to L.A.

Unfortunately, when it comes to healthy eating and weight release, this logic seems to go out the window. Too often we head off, not sure of our starting point or of our final destination. Sure, we know we want to lose weight, but that's like saying we want to go to Canada without indicating whether you want to go to Vancouver or Toronto. Without entering the exact coordinates of your starting location and your final destination, you'll end up just about anywhere.

So, that's where we'll begin today. Knowing your starting coordinates will allow you to enter a starting point into your GPS.

Now that you know where you want to go, you've got to know the coordinates of your starting point. Today, you're going to gather a baseline based on where you currently are in with your action step(s).

On day two, you allowed the Lord to show you one area in your relationship with food where you often break your boundaries. It could be decreasing your salt content, decreasing carbohydrate count, tracking your food, eliminating snacking, eating more vegetables, or drinking more water.

Based on what you identified, determine your specific starting point. For example:

If your stronghold is too much sodium, track how much sodium you consume in a day.

If your stronghold is too much sugar, track how much sugar you consume in a day.

If your stronghold is too many calories, track how many calories you're consuming per day.

If you consume certain foods late at night, identify what it is you're doing that leads you to eat at night.

If your stronghold is coffee, fat, or some other trigger food, identify just how much you're consuming and at what times.

If you're saying, "I hate tracking, it takes too much time." Or "Yeah, I used to track my food before", remember that the goal is not to track your food. The goal is to achieve your healthy weight so that you can achieve optimal health. So until you've achieved your goal, recognize that there is something that you don't know. Stay committed to doing what it takes until you've achieved your healthy weight. Don't worry about doing it every day, only focus on today. And like a good scientist, the purpose of tracking is to collect the necessary data to teach you something you did not know.

Tracking allows you to take responsibility for your relationship with food instead of just wondering why you can't ever get a foothold on the problem.

Tips for Tracking

To begin, don't restrict what you're eating. You want to get an accurate picture of what you're eating, so this is not the time to impress yourself with your good eating habits. Eat as you normally would.

1. Use a tracking app such as Myfitnesspal, Loseit, or Sparkpeople.

2. Keep it simple. Although you want to be as honest as possible, don't be too concerned with the exact item. Don't stress about whether you ate 13 or 14 almonds. The simpler you keep it, the higher the likelihood that you will continue to do it consistently.

3. Keep a journal. In addition to tracking your food, also keep a journal to help you understand some of your motivation around what you ate.

Other helpful things to pay attention to are:

What. What kinds of foods are you consuming specifically? For example, if you consume too much sugar, is it one, or two specific trigger foods? If it's fat, is it from nuts, meats, or fast foods?

Where (Location). Where are you eating the offensive foods? Are you consuming it standing, or in front of the TV? Is it linked to a specific location?

Who. Who do you eat the offensive food with? Are there specific people that sabotage you? Are there people who support you to eat healthfully?

When. What time do you consume the food(s)? Do you eat late at night?

Why. Why did you eat what you ate? Were you really hungry? Was it true hunger? Was there a specific emotion that triggered it?

How. How did you feel after you ate the trigger food? Were you bloated? Satisfied? How did you feel an hour later? How did you feel the next morning?

Chances are you will be shocked at what you discover when you begin tracking. As humans, we tend to underestimate our short-comings and overestimate our accomplishments. You'll probably notice the same pattern when it comes to tracking.

Remember that whether you track or not, your body will be tracking everything you eat, so you might as well get real with yourself. If you're currently tracking, are you seeing the benefits of this exercise? If not, then it might be time to tighten things up as you focus on this one specific action that continually sabotages you. Remember, you can't manage what you don't measure.

Action

Just for today, using an app like Myfitnesspal or another tracking app of your choice, track at a minimum the stronghold that you identified on day one. Gather as much information as you can about your stronghold.

Reflect

1. Read Proverbs 4:7 again. The Hebrew word David uses for "get wisdom" is "qana". It means to buy wisdom like a transaction. There is a price to pay if you want God's wisdom. Are you willing to pay the price for it? What do you need to sacrifice in order to obtain God's wisdom?

2. _____
   _____
   _____
   _____

   Where do you lack wisdom when it comes to healthy eating? Take time today and pray for wisdom.

   _____
   _____
   _____
   _____

3. What do you notice as you track the offensive food or habit?

   _____
   _____
   _____
   _____

Prayer

"Lord, I thank You for this process. Teach me what I need to know about food to best take care of my body. Food is Your medicine and I want to learn how to use it to heal and nourish my body. Help me be honest with myself about what I eat. I want results, but if I'm being honest I want to continue to enjoy food and I don't want to feel like I'm spending all my time counting calories and becoming obsessed. I want this process to be simple. I know it will take work and I'm ready for that, but I don't want it to be over-complicated. So help me, Lord, to do what I need to do now, so I don't have to keep falling into the same cycles of unhealthy eating. I thank You for what You are doing in my life and for how You are changing me. In Jesus' Name, Amen."

My Prayer

_____

_____

_____

_____

_____

_____

_____

_____

_____

Additional Scriptures

"'Surely not, Lord!' Peter replied. 'I have never eaten anything impure or unclean.' The voice spoke to him a second time, 'Do not call anything impure that God has made clean.'" ~Acts 10:14-15

"For physical training is of some value, but godliness has value for all things, holding promise for both the present life and the life to come." ~1 Timothy 4:8

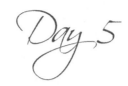

Walking in the Spirit

Scripture Reflection

"So I say, walk by the Spirit, and you will not gratify the desires of the flesh." ~Galatians 5:16

Devotion

I'm fascinated by how the brain works! I geek out in understanding neuroscience. The more I learn, the more I'm in awe of God's awesome creativity and supreme power.

It's from my verrrrryyyyy basic understanding of neuroscience that I've come to learn that there are three networks of the brain. For simplicity's sake, let's call them our lizard brain (the unconscious, automatic and most primitive part), the monkey brain(the emotional, irrational aspect fueled by fear and desire), and the human brain (the most conscious, rational, and logical aspect). It's our human brain that connects with God's Spirit.

Without the power of the Holy Spirit, we spend most of our time being led around by our monkey brain. It wants what it wants, when it wants it, and does not consider the consequences. When we're walking in the Spirit, we are able to exercise our human brain to subdue our flesh and calm our fears.

So what does that have to do with healthy eating and cravings?

In a fairly recent study[1] investigators found that when they temporarily decreased activity to the human brain—the brain which is responsible for self-control—study participants were drawn to high-calorie snacks and reported stronger urges to eat. This means that when you suppress the logical, rational aspect of your brain, it will act like your emotional, irrational brain, eating foods that it knows are not nutritious. So basically, science confirms what the Bible has taught us all along! We need the mind of Christ to keep us from falling into temptation.

We have two options: we can try to spend our time fighting our monkey brain (our sin nature) by making up a bunch of rules, trying to convince and discipline ourselves and make ourselves be better. But we only have to look at our past history to see that this is a losing proposition. The second option is to walk in the Spirit.

When we walk in the Spirit, we will make healthy food choices and not give in to our cravings.

How can you apply this principle to your healthy eating journey? Here are some tips to quiet your monkey brain and engage your human brain:

- Wake up and commit your day to the Lord. Ask Him to put a watch over your mouth.
- Pray before you eat each meal; pray for the spirit of self-control and that you will be satisfied.
- Spend time in the Word.
- Give praise and thanks to God in all situations and circumstances.

---

1   https://neurosciencenews.com/neuroscience-food-cravings-9598/#:~:text=The%20investigators%20found%20that%20when,urges%20to%20eat%20them%20than

- Get quiet. Before you eat, take some time and get quiet before the Lord— even if it's just a couple of seconds.

- Breathe. When you're losing a grip on your boundaries, take a deep breath in and invite the Holy Spirit.

Action

Make a list of habits and spiritual disciplines you will practice to keep your monkey brain from wanting to sabotage your commitment to healthy eating. **JUST FOR TODAY**, practice one of the spiritual disciplines when you notice your monkey brain wanting to sabotage your actions (specifically the one you committed to on day tw).

Reflect

1. Reflect on the role of your monkey brain as you think of all of the illogical and emotional thoughts that keep you from taking action and eating healthy. How does your monkey brain convince you to stray from your plans? What does it tell you?

   _____

   _____

   _____

   _____

2. When you're walking in the Spirit, your human brain is not easily led astray and you're able to make wise decisions that support your health. What will your human brain do when your needy monkey brain wants to start running the show?

_____

_____

_____

_____

Prayer

"Dear Lord, I thank You for reminding me that it is only when I walk in Your Spirit that I will not give rise to my flesh. As I walk out this journey of healthy eating, I keep my eyes and my mind fixed on You. I know that is the only way to win the battle for my mind. As sin is always knocking at my door, I know that it is only You that can rescue me from this body of death. Thank You for creating me so wonderfully, intricately, and complexly! I give you all glory, honor, and praise. In Your Name I pray, Amen!"

My Prayer

_____

_____

_____

_____

_____

_____

_____

_____

_____

Additional Scriptures

"Jesus said to them, 'I am the bread of life; whoever comes to me shall not hunger, and whoever believes in me shall never thirst.'" ~John 6:35

" Do not love the world or anything in the world. If anyone loves the world, love for the Father[a] is not in them. 16 For everything in the world—the lust of the flesh, the lust of the eyes, and the pride of life—comes not from the Father but from the world." ~1 John 2: 15

"So this is the principle I have discovered: When I want to do good, evil is right there with me." ~Romans 7:21

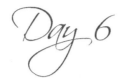

Brain vs Physical Hunger

Scripture Reflection

"Enter by the narrow gate. For the gate is wide and the way is easy that leads to destruction, and those who enter by it are many. For the gate is narrow and the way is hard that leads to life, and those who find it are few."
~Matthew 7:13-14 ESV

Devotion

Hunger can be classified in a variety of ways, ranging from taste hunger (wanting food just because you got a taste of it and want more), to practical hunger (having to eat during your lunch break because it's your designated time), to emotional hunger (driven by your emotions), to physical hunger (indicated by the growling tummy). This last one is the only type of hunger that comes from your physical body. It's triggered physiologically by your body's need for nutrients. We'll classify this as **'physical hunger'**. If you remember our three brains, this comes from our lizard brain.

Taste, practical, and emotional hunger come from either our lizard brain or our monkey brain when it tells you things like, "pack a snack with you in case you get hungry (lizard)," "oh, that cake looks so good, I want it (monkey)," or "I'm so mad, I need some wine (monkey)!" Impulses to eat are triggered from one of these sources of hunger we'll refer to as **'brain hunger'**, and it's the main reason for excess weight as we respond to our social cravings.

We live in a world where we could literally go for years without ever experiencing real physical hunger. Food is readily available everywhere, so we've become conditioned to eat just because it's there.

Because of our misuse of food, we've become afraid of hunger. Like a drug addict without their fix, you may feel panic set in when you are hungry and are not near to a food source. Or maybe, eating is so routine and habitual that you don't even think about it—you just eat.

But what if, on occasion, you learned to face your fears about hunger. What if you confronted hunger head on (or should I say mouth on). What if you learned to accept that hunger is nothing to panic about; it's not a crisis, or an emergency. Like feeling hot, cold, or tired, feeling hungry is uncomfortable, but there's a lot that we can learn instead of always giving in to our hunger. All of this is under the control of our third brain (human brain) as we walk in the spirit.

Learning to take control of your hunger instead of it controlling you will go a long way to help you stay on track with your healthy eating plan.

Imagine how much healthier you would be if you were no longer held hostage by your hunger.

If you did not give in to your cravings.

If you did not eat to pacify your feelings.

If you realized you were not hungry during your scheduled lunch hour at work.

If you decided not to have your usual dessert after dinner.

These are all choices that we make everyday, but too often we're not aware that we have a say in the matter of what, when, and how we eat. We've been led to believe that we have no power over our hunger, but that's a lie.

When you develop the practice of not always giving in to your hunger, you will feel so much more free.

Jesus teaches us about the power of choices that are often not popular and are *difficult*. In fact, Jesus warns us that when we go with the flow and give in to what we feel, it leads to destruction. Will you make the right choice today? Remember, it's just hunger. Like a loud plane passing overhead, the sensation will pass. As you learn to get in touch with occasionally going hungry, you'll get back in touch with your body's actual (not emotional) need for food, take back control over your own body, and enjoy your food that much more when you do eat.

To be clear, this does not mean that you're going to starve yourself or wait until you're completely famished, but merely to not pay attention to every "vague feeling" you experience between meals.

If you're not sure, an effective strategy to distinguish between brain hunger and physical hunger is the apple test. If you feel hungry between meals, ask yourself: "Would I eat vegetables or an apple?" If the answer is no, chances are you're probably not truly hungry.

Action

Just for today, you're going to experience what it feels like to be physically hungry. Start by letting yourself get physically hungry between meals. Wait until you feel the physical sensation of hunger before you eat. If you don't snack between meals, then eat one of your meals so that you still feel a bit of hunger.

When you feel hunger today, try to delay eating. Stop and pay attention to what you're eating and journal. Write down what you're feeling physically, mentally, and even emotionally. Notice if it's physical hunger or brain hunger, and journal where in your body you're experiencing the feelings.

Lastly, pay attention to your response when you begin to eat. Try to remain calm and relaxed. Pray before you eat and thank God for each bite, paying attention not to shovel the food into your mouth. Notice if you enjoy your food even more, being mindful not to overeat. Journal your experience.

Reflect

1. What factors determine your decisions to eat or not to eat? Are these factors based on your choice, circumstances, or something else? (Examples could include peer pressure, special events and celebrations, emotions such as loneliness, boredom, stress, or guilt.)

    _____

    _____

    _____

    _____

2. Do you feel like you have power to control what and when you eat, and the confidence and courage to maintain your boundaries? If not, ask the Lord to fill you with His power and authority to make good choices.

    _____

    _____

    _____

    _____

3. What would your life look like if you had power over
   your hunger? How would that look different from the
   decisions that you make each day around food?

_____

_____

_____

_____

Prayer

"Lord, I thank You that through Your strength I have the
power to choose when and what I will eat. Eating has become
so automatic for me that I no longer feel like I even have that
choice. In You I am strong. In You I choose the narrow gate. In
You I choose life over death and blessings over curses. In You I
choose to eat when I decide, not when my hunger dictates. In
You I choose what I will eat and where I eat, and will not allow
anything or anyone to make that decision for me. In Your Holy
Name, I pray! Amen."

My Prayer

_____

_____

_____

_____

_____

_____

_____

Additional Scriptures

"And do not get drunk with wine, for that is debauchery, but be filled with the Spirit." ~Ephesians 5:18

"But I say, walk by the Spirit, and you will not gratify the desires of the flesh." ~Galatians 5:16

"For to set the mind on the flesh is death, but to set the mind on the Spirit is life and peace." ~Romans 8:6

"No temptation has overtaken you that is not common to man. God is faithful, and he will not let you be tempted beyond your ability, but with the temptation, he will also provide the way of escape, that you may be able to endure it." ~1 Corinthians 10:1

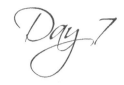

Week 1 Summary

Scripture Reflection

"Give thanks to the LORD, for he is good; his love endures forever." ~Psalm 107:1

Congratulations on completing your first week of *Healthy Eating, God's Way*!

Every six days you will take some time to recap, reflect, on what you have learned so far.

1. Recap

Which action step will you be recommitting to the Lord? How is it making a difference in your life so far? Recap what new insights you have learned this past week.

2. Reflect

Journal what the Holy Spirit is showing you so far. How will this new habit help you align with God's best for you?

3. Pray

Commit this next week to the Lord. Rest in Him and allow Him to give you the spirit of self-control and discipline.

Day 8

Planning for Success

Scripture Reflection

"The soul of a lazy man desires, and has nothing; But the soul of the diligent shall be made rich." ~Proverbs 13:4

Devotion

Why is it that one day we can feel so convicted and confident in our abilities and the next day we feel like we're right back to where we started? One day we declare, *"My plan is working. I feel so good and I have so much energy; I'm going to eat like this everyday."* Then 24 hours later, you wonder what happened to that confident, inspired warrior who made those vows. How do things change so quickly?

Remember our conversation about our three brains? We talked about the emotional monkey brain, sage human brain, and who can forget our efficient lizard brain. It's our subconscious lizard brain that manages all of our body functions, and it has one main function: survival. It's this survival instinct that's always telling us to conserve energy and take it easy. To put it bluntly, we're inherently lazy by nature[2].

This means that if we're not intentional, we will always take the path of least resistance. It's called efficiency and it's part of our make-up dating back to our hunting and gathering days when

2   https://time.com/4027942/lazy-walking-exercise/

preserving our energy was a matter of life or death. Fortunately, our hunter/gatherer days are long behind us and now food is abundant, so we no longer need to conserve energy. In fact, the opposite is now true. The over-abundance of food means that we have to move our bodies even more to compensate for the excess of food. We have to work to not overeat, but as you probably already recognized this will require that we walk in the Spirit to accomplish this great feat that our flesh is fighting against.

We have to be mindful of continually practicing healthy habits, otherwise we'll keep reverting to old habits. To eat healthy we need to be intentional, diligent, and proactive if we are going to be consistent in our efforts. We need to diligently and consistently plan and remain proactive.

As we've already discovered, the downside of our lizard brain is that it likes to take the path of least resistance. BUT, the upside of our lizard brain is that it likes to take the path of least resistance! We can use this to our favor by creating habits that we turn over to our lizard brain. Our lizard brain likes to automate functions, which is amazing because once your behaviors become automatic they will happen day in and day out without much thought or effort.

Imagine waking up each day and eating nutritious foods effortlessly without having to talk yourself into it or forcing yourself. Just like you walk into a dark room and turn on the light without thinking about it, that's the power of your lizard brain!

So what are the steps required for you to automate your action step? Let's learn how to turn it over to our lizard brain so we can "set it and forget it."

Action

Just for today, plan out all the steps involved in order to automate your action step. Write out a detailed step by step plan. As you plan, be mindful of distractions that might interfere with your routine such as electronic devices or multi-tasking.

Example: If your action step is to track your food, your routine might be:

1. 12:00 P.M. - Walk into the kitchen
2. 12:20 P.M. - Sit at the table
3. 12:21 P.M. - Pray
4. 12:22 P.M. - Eat lunch
5. 12:40 P.M. - Enter your food intake into Myfitnesspal. com
6. 12:42 P.M. - Wash up dishes

If you will be practicing your habit multiple times each day, start with just one.

Reflect

1. Review all the situations and circumstances that led you to stop practicing your action step. List them and write out what you will do if the situation arises. Example: For example, If I've set my calories limit for the day and I'm invited out to dinner, I will look ahead at the menu to pre-select a healthy choice that will fit within my boundaries.

    _____

    _____

    _____

    _____

2. Think of the last time you did not carry out your action step as you planned. What were the circumstances and what will you do differently next time?

_____

_____

_____

_____

3. Plan for contingencies. What does it take for you to maintain your goal each day consistently? Write it out specifically and methodically so that you can repeat it every day. Since my action step is to maintain 100 grams of carbohydrates here's my example:

- In order to maintain my action step, each day I will plan out what 100 grams of carbohydrates looks like the day prior.

- I will make sure that I have the foods on hand and will prepare any necessary foods so that I don't get too hungry and eat whatever I want.

- If I eat beyond my allotted portion, I will cut it back at the next meal or eliminate one of my snacks.

_____

_____

_____

_____

Prayer

"Lord, I see that I'm always reverting to my old habits. I often look for the easiest way, the fastest way, and the cheapest way sometimes and it rarely works out well. I've made a commitment, finally laying down this stronghold. I know that it can only happen when I walk step-by-step with You, so continue to lead me and I will follow You. Please help me be diligent in my planning; without a plan, I keep back-sliding. Keep me mindful that everything I do is to glorify You. Your Word reminds me of all of the benefits of a diligent person, and I want that to be me. I want to experience all the fruits and benefits like courage, discipline, strength, and perseverance. In Your Name, I pray. Amen!"

My Prayer

_____

_____

_____

_____

_____

_____

_____

_____

Additional Scriptures

"Whatever you do, work at it with all your heart, as working for the Lord, not for human masters, since you know that you will receive an inheritance from the Lord as a reward. It is the Lord Christ you are serving." ~Colossians 3:23-24

"Let me hear Your lovingkindness in the morning; For I trust in You; Teach me the way in which I should walk; For to You I lift up my soul." ~Psalms 143:8 NIV

"The hand of the diligent will rule, But the lazy man will be put to forced labor." ~Proverbs 12:24

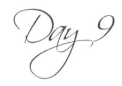

You Are What You Eat

Scripture Reflection

"Every moving thing that lives shall be food for you. And as I gave you the green plants, I give you everything."
~Genesis 9:3

Devotion

The question people most commonly ask me is, "What should I eat?" Or some version of the similar question which includes:

What diet is the right one for me—Keto, Paleo, LCHF, Mediterranean? Should I do intermittent fasting; and if so, how many hours and what should I eat when my eating window opens?

These are all fair questions, but they are not the right questions.

Truth is, most of us are not really looking for the healthiest way to eat when we ask these questions. We're really looking for the "hacks." We want the best, quickest, simplest, and most efficient way. Unfortunately, those are not always what's right for our bodies.

It does not matter whether you practice intermittent fasting, Keto, Paleo, or live solely on organic food. Healthy eating is an individual journey that will take time and practice. There really are no shortcuts, but you can learn the right approach to take. That's what you'll discover in this devotional and challenge.

So if you find yourself gaining weight, or even maintaining weight despite intermittent fasting and working out, if you have no idea how many calories you consume each day, if you have challenges with entitlement (you deserve it), or struggle with a spirit of rebellion, this book will teach you how to eat healthy despite not having the "perfect diet." What you will end up with is the perfect diet for you!

That will happen for you as you learn to understand your body and its caloric and emotional needs, your propensities and proclivities, your fear and limiting beliefs around food, and mostly your willingness to submit your health journey to the Lord.

You truly are what you eat. This can be both metaphorical and physical. Your amazing body takes the foods you eat and turns them into all parts of you. That's good news and bad news depending on what you eat. If you eat good food, your body will be healthy and strong. Conversely, if you eat garbage . . .

As you eat, your body breaks down foods into their chemical parts like macronutrients and micronutrients. Macronutrients are the structural components of our foods and they provide us with energy. They include carbohydrates, fats, and proteins. A very basic rule of thumb is to consume 33.3% of your daily calories from each of these groups.

Micronutrients are the vitamins, minerals, trace elements, phytochemicals, and antioxidants that are essential for good health. During this course, we're going to focus solely on macronutrients.

Carbohydrates

Carbohydrates include a big umbrella of foods ranging from chocolate bars to bread, pasta, fruits, grain products, starchy vegetables, beans, legumes, and juices. They include both junk foods (refined carbs) and nutritious foods (whole grains). Most of us eat too many refined carbohydrates and not enough complex carbohydrates such as beans, whole grains, and vegetables. If consuming 33.3% of your daily calories seems too low for you then maybe start by decreasing your current consumption by 20%.

Proteins

They do most of the work in cells and are required for the structure, function, and regulation of the body's tissues and organs. They are made up of twenty amino acids. Protein can be found in most foods, but the most concentrated forms can be found in meat, poultry, seafood, eggs, soy, beans, and nuts. They are more difficult for our bodies to break down than carbohydrates, so they keep you fuller longer. Most of us do not eat enough protein.

Fats

Fats are nutrients in food that the body uses to build cell membranes, assist in hormone production, and a lot of other important roles. Fat-containing foods are avocados, nuts and seeds, or animal fats such as butter. They are more difficult to break down in the body, so they leave you more satisfied than carbohydrates. Most of us eat too much bad fats found in processed foods and not enough good fats found in avocados and nuts.

Calories

A calorie is simply a measure of energy that you ingest in food. Carbohydrates, fats, and proteins combine to make up the majority of the number of calories you consume each day. The number of calories that you eat each day should be based on your activity level, metabolism, age, height, weight, and sex. On average, you need 1,600–2,000 per day.

Today, you're going to start this process by getting a snapshot of how many calories you consumed yesterday and how many of them were derived from carbohydrates, fats, and proteins.

Action

Take the time today and calculate your daily caloric needs if you don't already know it, and compare it to your current caloric consumption. What is the difference?

If you have not already done so, set up a MyFitnessPal (myfitnesspal.com) account or another tracking tool that you prefer and begin tracking your food.

To determine your daily caloric needs, go to:

https://www.myfitnesspal.com/tools/bmr-calculator
(go to additional resources).

My Fitness Pal Training Video:
weightlossgodsway.com/myfitnesspal

Reflect

1. Are you willing to let go of finding the perfect diet and discover the right way to eat for your body?

_____

_____

2. Do you have a good understanding of the difference between carbohydrates, fats, and proteins? Select a few from each category that are right for your unique body.

_____

_____

_____

_____

3. Which of the three macronutrients (carbs, fats, or proteins) are you most challenged with maintaining (either in excess, or deficiency), and what will you do to increase or decrease your consumption of them?

_____

_____

_____

_____

Prayer

"Lord, I thank You that You continue to challenge me so that I can grow stronger in You. With every challenge and every temptation, I call on You and call Your Name. I know that You will always answer me. Satisfy me with Your love. When I feel like I need more food, more satisfaction, more love, remind me that it is all found in You and You alone. Remind me that my food is to the will of my Father. Remind me of how little food I actually need each day and renew my taste buds so that they enjoy wholesome and nutritious foods. Give me a disdain for feeling like I need to feel stuffed. I declare that I eat within my boundaries and am satisfied. In Jesus' Name, Amen."

My Prayer

_____

_____

_____

_____

_____

_____

_____

_____

Additional Scriptures

"Do you not know that your body is a temple of the Holy Spirit who is in you, whom you have received from God? You are not your own." ~1 Corinthians 6:19

"Let not sin therefore reign in your mortal body, that ye should obey it in the lusts thereof." ~Romans 6:12

"Those who belong to Christ Jesus have crucified the flesh with its passions and desires." ~Galatians 5:24

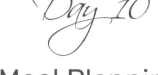

Meal Planning

Scripture Reflection

"Suppose one of you wants to build a tower. Won't you first sit down and estimate the cost to see if you have enough money to complete it?" ~Luke 14:28

Devotion

So much of our challenges with healthy eating would be solved if we took the time to plan. That's because when we don't have a plan we let our emotions decide what we should eat (monkey brain) or we default to high fat, high sugar food because that's what our bodies will default to for survival (lizard brain). But with proper planning, we can make wise choices that keep us eating healthfully, and the best part about it is that we don't have to give it much thought. We simply eat what we planned.

Unfortunately, most of us get completely overwhelmed with the thought of planning out an entire week of eating—especially when we don't even know what we'll be eating for our next meal let alone six days from now. Secondly, many women often tell me that they rarely eat what they planned because they don't feel like eating that particular food when the day arrives. To that I would say, if you're truly serious about wanting to release your excess weight, put your feelings aside and eat what you've prepared. The question will always come down to, "How bad do you want it?"

With that not so gracious but honest answer, let's look at some do's and don'ts of meal planning.

- Commit to it! It may sound simple, but if you've never actually parked your behind in a chair with the intention of planning your meals, it might seem overwhelming. So the first step is to make up your mind and commit to the process.

- We get overwhelmed because we're busy focusing on low carb, low calorie, low fat options that leave us feeling like we have no choice. If something happens to be high fat, simply have less of it.

- Schedule a consistent day and time each week that you will plan, shop, and prepare your meals. For example, I begin planning on Friday, shop on Saturday, and cook on Sundays.

- Print out a weekly calendar and start by filling in the blanks with foods that you automatically eat (morning smoothie, taco Tuesday, etc.)

- Brainstorm a list of foods that you enjoy. Break it into breakfasts, lunches, snacks and dinners, proteins, carbs, good fats and veggies, and plug those in your calendar first.

- Take an inventory of what foods are currently in your freezer or fridge that you can incorporate into your meals.

- Measure your food using zip lock bags, containers, spoons, the palm of your hand, or invest in an inexpensive scale.

- Keep it simple. Select 1-2 meats and change it up. Ground beef can be used for chili, burritos, shepherd's pie, and a pasta dish.

- Don't feel you have to be super-creative and come up with different meals everyday—change it slightly from one night to the next.
- Visit Pinterest for meal planning ideas.
- Start where you're at. If the prospect of planning all your meals seems too overwhelming, can you start with just dinners?
- Try a meal kit company like Hello Fresh, Chef's Plate, or Good Food.
- Try meal-preparing apps such as Yummly or Mealtime.
- Keep it simple by having theme days such as Meatless Mondays, Taco Tuesday, or Soup on Saturdays.
- Invest in proper storage containers.
- Double or triple batch recipes to save time and energy.
- Don't be afraid to eat the same thing a few days in a row.
- Invest in a slow cooker or Instant-Pot so you can throw food in and go about your chores without having to constantly watch over your meal.
- Pair fresh salads with already prepared foods from the grocery store, such as rotisserie chicken.

Action

Today you're going to plan out your meal for the entire day, if you have not already done so. Start with dinner since that's usually the most challenging. First think of your choice of protein and a small starch if any at all, then do your best to fill up your plate with vegetables. Also plan what time you will be eating your meals.

Reflect

1. What keeps you from meal planning? Is it intimidating or overwhelming?

   _____

   _____

   _____

   _____

2. How do you think meal planning would benefit your health?

   _____

   _____

   _____

   _____

3. What is one thing that you can do to move you closer to developing the discipline of planning your meals?

   _____

   _____

   _____

   _____

Prayer

"Father God, we thank You for creating our bodies. We thank You, Jesus, for Your great wisdom in giving us a blueprint of how to care for Your temple. We thank You for Your love and mercy. God, we want to honor You with our bodies and our minds. Help us to learn how to be more efficient with our time. If there are areas in our schedule that need to be reevaluated, then reveal that to us. We remain willing to change for You and be all that You want us to be. In Jesus' Name, Amen."

My Prayer

Additional Scriptures

"Commit your actions to the Lord, and your plans will succeed." ~Proverbs 16:3 (NLT)

"Careful planning puts you ahead in the long run; hurry and scurry puts you further behind." ~Proverbs 21:5 (MSG)

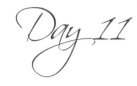

The Importance of Water

Scripture Reflection

"But whoever drinks of the water that I will give him will never be thirsty again. The water that I will give him will become in him a spring of water welling up to eternal life."
~John 4:14

Devotion

What's the Big Deal About Water?

The Earth is 70% water. Your body is 80% water. It stands to reason that water is essential for life. Water is the body's transportation vehicle. It is used to move nutrients to the 100 trillion cells in your body, to move waste and toxins from your cells to your kidneys then out of your body, and it helps your body eliminate fat.

How Much Water Should You Drink?

Drink half an ounce for every pound of your weight ... every day.

Example:

If you weigh 150 pounds, you would drink 75 ounces per day or nine cups of water (75 divided by 8 oz).

If you weigh 200 pounds, you would drink 100 ounces per day or 12 cups of water (100 divided by 8 oz).

Benefits of Drinking Water

- Drinking water is great for fat loss. It removes byproducts of fat from your body, it leaves you feeling full so that you don't eat as much, it reduces hunger, it boosts your metabolism, and it's fat and calorie-free.

- Since your brain is mostly water, drinking it helps with focus, concentration, and alertness. Drinking water will give you a quick and healthy energy boost when you're feeling tired.

- Drinking water eliminates toxins. It helps your body get rid of waste through urination, which reduces the risk of kidney stones and UTIs (urinary tract infections).

- Water can help reduce stomach acidity.

- It maintains regularity.

- Constipated? Drinking your recommended water intake each day is a simple way to ease chronic constipation. Try drinking a glass of water as soon as you wake up to help stimulate bowel movements.

- Water is a natural headache remedy. It helps to relieve and prevent headaches (migraines and back pain, too!) which are commonly caused by dehydration.

- It prevents cramps and sprains.

- Proper hydration helps keep joints lubricated and muscles more elastic so joint pain is less likely.

- What they found was that the greater the water consumption, the better the mood. Tension, depression, and confusion scores went down when water intake went up.

- Drinking water improves physical performance. If we do not stay hydrated, physical performance can suffer.

- Dehydration can have a noticeable effect if you lose as little as 2% of your body's water content. If you feel fatigued when exercising for a long time, it's a good idea to drink some water.

- If you want to perform optimally when exercising, make sure you're well hydrated.

- Drinking water can help you lose weight. This is due to the fact that water can increase satiety and boost your metabolic rate.

- Water aids in circulation.

- Over half of your blood consists of a substance called plasma, which is about 90% water. Plasma carries blood cells around your body to where they're needed, helps maintain healthy blood pressure, and keeps your body temperature under control.

- Without enough water, your blood will become thicker and more concentrated. This means your heart has to work all that much more to pump blood to the entire body.

- If you feel tired during the day, instead of going for a cup of coffee which will actually dehydrate you try drinking some water instead. That lethargic and tired feeling you experience can be a sign of dehydration, which coffee will only provide a temporary boost for. [3]

Action

Using the formula above, be intentional today about drinking your required amount of water. What did you notice? What

---

3   https://www.mindbodygreen.com/articles/does-coffee-count-as-water

challenges did you experience? What impact did it have on your appetite? Journal your insights.

Reflect

1. How much water do you currently drink? How much should you be drinking?

    _____

    _____

    _____

2. What comparisons can you make with spiritual water and drinking water?

    _____

    _____

    _____

3. What benefits are you most looking forward to as you increase your water consumption?

    _____

    _____

    _____

Prayer

"Dear Lord, I thank You for providing us with fresh water to drink today and every day. Let me never take this precious commodity for granted. It's amazing how, just like You, water is so essential for life. Just like with You, we can't go for very long without water. So every time I drink it, remind me of You. Help me to stay hydrated each day and help me learn to love water. It is life! In Jesus' Name I pray. Amen."

My Prayer

_____

_____

_____

_____

_____

_____

_____

Additional Scriptures

"This is the one who came by water and blood—Jesus Christ. He did not come by water only, but by water and blood. And it is the Spirit who testifies because the Spirit is the truth."
~1 John 5:6

"Then will I sprinkle clean water upon you, and ye shall be clean: from all your filthiness, and from all your idols, will I cleanse you." ~Ezekiel 36:25

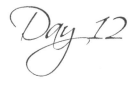

Feel Your Feelings and Feed Your Hunger

Scripture Reflection

"Be angry and do not sin; do not let the sun go down on your anger, and give no opportunity to the devil." ~Ephesians 4:26-27

Devotion

Emotional eating plays a big factor in our "inability'" to eat healthfully.

Experts estimate that 80% of overeating is emotional. I don't know who those experts are since this is one of those statistics that gets thrown around the health and wellness world, but my own life can attest to the relative accuracy. After my first meal of the day (which is around noon), most of what I eat is usually out of boredom, habit, anxiety or, if it's the weekend, entitlement. You know the feeling: "I've had a hard week so I deserve to eat whatever I want on the weekend," or "I've been good all week so I deserve a treat."

My body feels healthiest when I eat a fairly large meal at lunch, a light snack a few hours later, followed by a very light meal around 5:00 P.M. Yet, as I write this, my daily diet is a far cry from that. I've accepted where I am on my journey, believing that one day I will get there. Admittedly, everything else outside of those three meals is emotional.

Emotional eating is when we eat in response to our feelings regardless of whether we're hungry or not, and/or when we use food as a tool or coping mechanism to either numb pain or to feel better. It's the automatic and subconscious responses that make our emotions so powerful and dangerous. In this case, the monkey brain may have initiated the sequence of events to eat, but then turned it over to the lizard brain once it got habituated and became routine. Remember, anything that becomes a habit is turned over to the lizard brain, which runs on autopilot.

I remember when my doctor told me that I was borderline diabetic. You would think that would have been enough for me to change, but as much as I tried I still could not stop myself from bingeing on sweets.

Why couldn't I stop, even though I knew that this could lead to irreparable hardship? Because I was not conscious of what triggered my emotional eating, and even when I did gain awareness, my willpower was no match for my feelings and emotions. I've spent most of my adult life learning how to stuff my uneasy feelings back down with food so I don't have to feel them. Like a pacifier, a large population of society and I use food to comfort us, or make us feel better when we're stressed, angry, lonely, bored, frustrated, or a multitude of other emotions that we experience.

But it's not supposed to be this way. Our goal is to learn how to feel our feelings and feed our hunger instead of feeding our feelings and refusing to feel hunger.

Know this, there's a reason you choose to feed your feelings instead of feeling them. Because these feelings are painful!

Their roots are grounded in discomfort, pain, or trauma. And why on Earth would we want to experience pain?

Except you probably know all too well that "feeding" it with food does not take away the pain permanently. The benefit, if you want to call it that, lasts only as long as the taste of the food swirling around in your mouth. Soon after that comes the guilt and shame, if you're conscious of your patterns. If you're on autopilot, then you may not even be aware of why you're eating when you're not hungry.

In Ephesians 4:26-27, Paul is using the emotion of anger, but we can apply any emotion that leads us to eat. He is saying that we can feel our feelings, but we don't have to act on the feeling. We can feel anger, frustration, sadness, or stress and NOT eat to numb those unwanted feelings. As we learn how to stop allowing our emotions to lead our behavior, we keep the enemy from having control of our health.

Today you will pay attention to the emotions that dictate and sabotage your health. Then you will discover how to let the Word of God dictate your actions, choices, decisions, and behaviors. It's the only way to true healing and freedom.

Action

Just for today, you will track everything you eat. If you're using a tracking app then rewrite it in your journal, placing either an "H" for hungry, or "E" for emotional beside everything you eat. If you're not hungry, assume it's emotional. Then write out what the emotion is that led you to eat. If you already track that's great, but if you don't, remember that you only have to do it for today.

Reflect

1. What are the recurrent emotions that lead you to eat when you're not hungry?

   _____

   _____

   _____

2. What does Paul mean when he says to not let the sun go down on your anger? How can you apply that principle to your healthy eating journey?

   _____

   _____

   _____

3. What are some biblical strategies that you will use to help you manage your emotions? (Prayer, declarations, active practice, etc.)

   _____

   _____

   _____

Prayer

Dear Lord, thank You that You are so much greater than my feelings!! I've been dragged around by them into all kinds of situations that have left me full of shame and guilt. In many ways, God, I have made my feelings my Lord and let them rule over me in the place that You belong as my only authority NOT my moods or feelings and NOT fear of other people's opinions. I've done what I hate so many times because of my feelings, usually trying to avoid the ones that feel awful but sometimes just to enjoy the ones that feel great. Please forgive me, Lord!

Today, I am trusting in Your unconditional love and in the knowledge that You are so much greater than my feelings! Help me please to trust in You when I start to feel tempted to let my feelings be my boss. Reassure me in my hour (or split second!) of need that Your ways are so much greater than mine, and that includes my feelings. Give me the patience to pause before acting on them, allowing them to just be. You are truly awesome, God! In Jesus' Name, Amen.

My Prayer

_____

_____

_____

_____

_____

_____

_____

_____

_____

_____

Additional Scriptures

"For the Spirit God gave us does not make us timid, but gives us power, love and self-discipline." ~2 Timothy 1:7

"Therefore, there is now no condemnation for those who are in Christ Jesus." ~Romans 8:1

"Therefore, since we have been justified by faith, we have peace with God through our Lord Jesus Christ." ~Romans 5:1

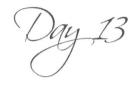

Reasons or Results

Scripture Reflection

"I have no one to help me into the pool when the water is stirred. While I am trying to get in, someone else goes down ahead of me." ~John 5:7

Overview

I often hear women say, "I don't like tracking because it takes too much time." Or "Planning my meals takes too much work." My response is always the same: If you believe it's worth it, you'll find a way. If it's not, you'll find an excuse. As harsh as it may sound, that's the bottom line.

If you look at anyone who is successful at anything, you'll see their familiar story. They put in the time, they did the work, they made sacrifices, they pushed past their comfort zone, learning how to submit their struggles to the Lord. Sure, there might be a bit of genetics involved, but they had to nurture those gifts in order to get their results. So why do we think it should be any different when it comes to healthy eating?

Excuse-making is a defensive or protective mechanism to justify our behaviors. So it's not enough to tell ourselves to just STOP making excuses; we need to identify what the fears and limiting beliefs are that keep us stuck in this pattern. As Dr Phil always says, "It's impossible to change what you don't acknowledge."

When Jesus asked the man at the pool if he wanted to be well, he responded with an excuse. Why would his first response be an excuse? We can only surmise that he had grown so tired and so weary that, where he once might have seen possibility, he now only saw pain; where he once saw healing, he only saw heartbreak. So his only logical response now was to give reasons for why what he wanted was no longer possible.

Like him, excuses can become our automatic responses—our new normal—instead of holding on to our hope, promise, or expectation. EXCUSES justify why what we want is not possible. EXPECTATIONS declare what is possible when they are aligned with God's plans for us.

Excuses keep us from taking responsibility for our lives and our health. They rob us of our personal power and leave us feeling helpless in our circumstances.

Today, take the time to identify why you sometimes make excuses. Don't focus on the exceptional circumstances like a death in the family or a serious injury. Look at the chronic excuses that you continually make and have probably been making for years. Give those to God in prayer and let Him show you that fear is at the root.

Action

Look at your action step and identify all of the excuses you make for why you don't carry it out. For example, if your action step is to walk you might say, "It's raining outside." "It's too cold or hot," "I don't have enough time". Pray about what the truth is behind the fear or limiting belief and then make a plan for what you will do in the event of the excuse. For example, if it's raining outside put on a workout video and exercise at home.

Reflect

1. Think of the last time you failed to practice your action step. What was the reason? What could you have done instead?

    _____

    _____

    _____

2. Identify up to three excuses you make that prevent you from reaching your healthy weight.

    _____

    _____

    _____

3. Share the biggest excuse you often make with your accountability partner and let them know what you will do the next time you hear yourself making that excuse.

    _____

    _____

    _____

Prayer

"Dear Lord, I thank You for helping me to understand that even though I have the freedom to eat whatever I want, it is not beneficial. I'm so grateful for boundaries that keep me safe and protected and I'm equally grateful for challenges that take me out of my comfort zone while keeping me safe in Your loving arms. Thank You for this challenge. It is just what I need at this season in my life where I need a breakthrough. Food continues to have this hold on me and I want it broken, Lord, in Your

Name. I do so well for a little while and then something happens and I find myself right back where I started. I know I'm making progress even though sometimes it does not feel like it. Prepare my heart and mind for this challenge. Help me to turn away from foods that are not good for me and help me to crave You instead of food. In Your Holy Name I pray. Amen!"

My Prayer

_____

_____

_____

_____

_____

_____

_____

_____

_____

_____

Additional Scriptures

"The heart is deceitful above all things and beyond cure. Who can understand it?" ~Jeremiah 17:9

"For we must all appear before the judgment seat of Christ, so that each one may receive what is due for what he has done in the body, whether good or evil." ~2 Cor 5:10

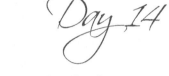

Day 14

Week 2 Summary

Scripture Reflection

"Give thanks to the LORD, for he is good; his love endures forever." ~Psalms 107:1

Congratulations on completing week 2!

As we wrap up this week, review what you've learned.

1. Recap

What new concepts or principles did you learn about healthy eating? Briefly recap that last six lessons and review any 'a-ha' moments or insights.

2. Reflect

Journal what the Holy Spirit has shown you this week. How many days did you successfully complete your action step?

3. Pray

Commit your week to the Lord. Rest in Him and continue to take it one day at a time. Don't worry about what you will eat tomorrow—focus on eating healthfully today.

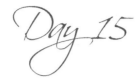

Moderate or Eliminate?

Scripture Reflection

*"But put on the Lord Jesus Christ, and make no provision for
the flesh, to gratify its desires." ~Romans 13:14*

Devotion

For years I touted the principle of moderation to all my clients.
And for the same amount of time, I also attempted to live by
this principle myself. "Everything in moderation," I used to say.
But I would always have a difficult time putting it into practice.
And because it was only with a few foods I never considered it
a serious problem, so the idea of giving up the offensive food
entirely never occurred to me.

Only after talking to client after client, and member after
member, did I realize that the famous 'everything in moderation'
principle was not gonna cut it for everyone. After digging a bit
deeper, I learned that for some people there is no such thing as
'just one bite'. And to complicate things even further, not only
are there certain people with addictive tendencies but there are
also addictive foods.

Let's explore the notion of addictive-prone people and addictive
foods.

Are You a Food Addict?

Like alcoholics or sexaholics, there is also an estimated over 70 million people world–wide[4] addicted to food. If you think it might be you, you can take the quiz here[5]. Food addicts will eat despite the negative consequences of weight gain or even a negative doctor's report.

The problem for food addicts is that once they consume the addictive food, the reward or pleasure center in the brain causes people to lose control of their impulses and overrides other signals that would otherwise say that you're full or satisfied. For food addicts there is no such thing as moderation, because they are unable to stop after just one bite of the trigger foods.

The Bliss Point

There are also certain combinations of foods that are specifically created to make us crave them, even when we're not hungry! For this, we can thank Howard Moskowitz, an American market researcher known for creating addictive flavor combinations that keep us overeating our favorite snack foods. He determined the exact combination of fat, sugar, and salt to excite our taste buds and override the brain's natural 'stop' signals. Ever notice that some of the most addictive foods are laden with high amounts of sugar, fat, and salt? He called this the 'bliss point', which is why we keep coming back for more even though our bodies are telling us to stop—sometimes even to the point of feeling literally sick!

In addition to food combinations of sugar, fat and salt, there may also be some 'trigger foods' that cause you to overeat. These are foods that 'One bite is too much and a thousand will

---

4   https://www.orlandosentinel.com/health/os-food-addiction-numbers-rising-20160902-story.html

5   https://www.foodaddicts.org/am-i-a-food-addict

never be enough' as the expression goes, when it comes to these genetically modified weapons of mass addiction!

To effectively release weight, those foods must be eliminated from your diet. Don't even mess around with them. The second it touches your lips, it will trigger a biochemical response that will render you powerless to that food—and good luck trying to stop yourself.

If you've determined that you're not a food addict but you're still not sure if you should moderate or eliminate, ask yourself this simple question: "Can I eat just one cookie (cake/chocolate, a handful of chips, nuts, etc.) and feel satisfied?"

If the answer is no, then those are your trigger foods and you need to eliminate them from your life.

If you are the type of person who can eat one cookie and stop, then keep on with your "everything in moderation" principle.

As Paul writes to the Christians in Rome, he urges them (and, by extension, us) to avoid those situations that will open the door to lead us to give in to our flesh.

We control our appetites, they do not control us. Let that be our gauge to tell whether we are walking in the Spirit or the flesh.

Action

Today, complete the food addicts questionnaire (foodaddicts. org/am-i-a-food-addict) and follow the post-assessment instructions. If you've determined that you're not a food addict, make a list of your trigger foods.

Reflect

1. What situations trigger you to overeat?

    _____
    _____
    _____

2. What happens to us spiritually as we give in to our flesh?

    _____
    _____
    _____

3. When was the last time you lost control after consuming a trigger food? What were the effects?

    _____
    _____
    _____

4. Like putting on a coat each day, how can you practically 'put on' the Lord Jesus Christ? (Romans 13:14)

    _____
    _____
    _____

Prayer

"Lord, I thank You that through Your strength, I walk in the Spirit. It is the only way that I will not give in to my cravings and desires. Sometimes I feel like a spoiled brat—I want what I want, when I want it, even though I know that it will only hurt me in the long run. Let me only seek Your best for me.

Strengthen me so I can resist the enemy when he tries to tempt me. And thank You in advance for always providing a way of escape. In Your Holy Name I pray! Amen."

My Prayer

_____

_____

_____

_____

_____

_____

_____

_____

_____

_____

Additional Scriptures

"And do not get drunk with wine, for that is debauchery, but be filled with the Spirit." ~Ephesians 5:18

"But I say, walk by the Spirit, and you will not gratify the desires of the flesh." ~Galatians 5:16

"For to set the mind on the flesh is death, but to set the mind on the Spirit is life and peace." ~Romans 8:6

"No temptation has overtaken you that is not common to man. God is faithful, and he will not let you be tempted beyond your ability, but with the temptation, he will also provide the way of escape, that you may be able to endure it." ~1 Corinthians 10:13

Day 16

Mindful Eating

Scripture Reflection

"The mind governed by the flesh is death, but the mind governed by the Spirit is life and peace." ~Romans 8:6

Devotion

The WeightLossGodsWay.com definition of mindful eating is the practice of paying attention to how the food we eat glorifies God. It is an awareness of how your food nourishes your body, soul, and spirit; an acknowledgment of God's role in the food we eat by giving Him thanks for it and a recognition that food is a gift from God.

If you've ever wolfed down a bag of Doritos or inhaled a pint of Häagen-Dazs, then you know how easy it is to disconnect our mind from our body and spirit as we eat.

Today you're going to begin reconnecting, and it starts by getting present to some of the thoughts swirling around in your mind about food. You see, we've fallen for so many of the lies of the enemy that we often eat without connecting the dots. Then we wonder why food continues to have its grip on us.

There's a dynamic interaction between our body, mind, and spirit which goes like this: spirits control our mind which in turn control our actions such as eating. So if your mind is focused on your flesh, your wants, your needs, your desires, your problems, then it will continue to struggle with making healthy food choices. But if your mind is focused on the Spirit, you will find peace and freedom.

As you continue to practice letting go by detaching and separating your feelings from present situations and circumstances today, you'll add another tool to your arsenal, called 'mindful eating'.

Here's how:

1. EAT SLOWLY

Ever heard the expression, 'speed kills'? This applies to the way you eat, too. Eating too quickly leads to poor digestion. Instead of shoveling food into your mouth (I'm guilty of this,) practice putting your fork down in between bites. Chew your food as much as possible—actually count it and see how many bites you can take before it's all gone. Aim for 20-30 chews.

2. PRACTICE EATING AT A TABLE

Do you eat while watching TV or standing around the kitchen island? Try making most meals (at least dinner) a special time for enjoyment and rest. Use nice dishes, drink out of a wine glass, and enjoy the entire dining experience.

3. GIVE THANKS

Give thanks for your food and for everyone involved in getting it to the table.

4. CHECK IN WITH YOUR BODY

How does the food you're eating make you feel? Did it satisfy you? Did it make you feel gassy or bloated or tired? If a certain food triggers a reaction, make a note of it and eliminate it from your diet. Foods should energize you and make you feel good after eating them.

5. AVOID EATING WHILE STRESSED, ARGUING, OR UPSET

Eating under stress promotes poor digestion. The stress also triggers a cortisol response which leads to overeating— especially non-nutritious foods.

6. UNDERSTAND HOW MUCH FOOD YOU'RE EATING

Mindful eating involves knowing the quality and quantity of the food you're eating. Are you eating 1,500 calories or 3,000 calories? Are you eating enough protein, calories, and fat at each meal? As you plan your meals, be mindful that you're giving your body the nutrition it needs.

7. ASK YOURSELF POWERFUL QUESTIONS

Why am I eating this? Will I regret this tomorrow? Am I being the best version of myself? How will eating this make me feel? Challenge yourself by asking yourself questions that will make you think.

8. PRACTICE SMILING WHEN EATING

Why? Because food is a gift from God. Every time you eat, see it as a eucharist to Him; it should bring a smile to your face. It might seem hokey, but I challenge you to give it a try.

Action

Today you will practice mindful eating by being intentional about what you eat. You will begin by properly plating your meal, moving slowly and relaxed as you prepare to eat. Start by thanking God for the meal and everything that went into getting the food to your table, including the truck drivers, store clerks, field workers, farmers, bakers, etc. Be sure you're sitting at a table instead of standing or eating on the run. Engage all of your senses as you eat. Notice the colors in your food. What does it smell like? Pay attention to the variety of textures. Enjoy all the different tastes—is it sweet, savoury, salty, or tangy? Then chew your food deliberately and slowly, taking your time to put your fork down between bites.

Reflect

1. What difference did it make when you ate mindfully? How would this practice improve your overall health?

   _____

   _____

   _____

   _____

2. What adjustments will you incorporate into your life to help with mindful eating?

   _____

   _____

   _____

   _____

3. What does 1 Peter 5:8 and Matthew 15:11 teach you about mindful eating?

   _____

   _____

   _____

   _____

Prayer

"Dear Lord, my mind is so full that I'm rarely mindful of what I'm eating. And when I am, it's because I'm usually feeling guilt or shame about eating something that I should not have. I so want to be free from the bondage of food! I don't want it taking up so much mental space in my mind. Teach me that food is not the enemy; change my relationship with food so I can see it as a gift from You. Help me to be mindful of what I put into my mouth and let me enjoy every morsel. I have Your mind, Lord, and it brings me peace and joy. So I thank You that I don't have to be a prisoner of my own thoughts. When I eat, when I go to work, when I walk around, I give it all to You as worship. I keep my mind fixed on You because You are the author and perfecter of my faith. In Your Name I pray. Amen!"

My Prayer

_____

_____

_____

_____

_____

_____

_____

_____

_____

Additional Scriptures

"Be sober [well balanced and self-disciplined], be alert and cautious at all times. That enemy of yours, the devil, prowls around like a roaring lion [fiercely hungry], seeking someone to devour."
~1 Peter 5:8

"Let this mind be in you, which was also in Christ Jesus."
~Philippians 2:5

"So here's what I want you to do, God helping you: Take your everyday, ordinary life—your sleeping, eating, going-to-work, and walking-around life—and place it before God as an offering." ~Romans 12:1

"We do this by keeping our eyes on Jesus, the champion who initiates and perfects our faith. Because of the joy awaiting him, he endured the cross, disregarding its shame. Now he is seated in the place of honor beside God's throne."
~Hebrews 12:2 NLT

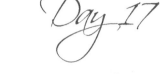

Should I Snack?

Scripture Reflection

"No temptation has overtaken you that is not common to man. God is faithful, and he will not let you be tempted beyond your ability, but with the temptation, he will also provide the way of escape, that you may be able to endure it." ~1 Corinthians 10:13

Devotion

One of the biggest myths to ever dominate the health world is that you should eat every few hours.

Heck, I was also guilty of advising clients to "eat every three to four hours to prevent your body from going into starvation mode." Like many other health professionals, that's what I was taught and truly believed.

Thus, the advent of a generation of people ignoring their body's hunger signals was born. Regardless of whether they were hungry or not, people ate; regardless of whether they were losing weight, they ate. After all, they did not want their body to go into starvation mode and stop burning calories.

Grocery shelves in the '60s and '70s began to stock snack foods in individual serving sizes for people on the go. We would never leave home without snacks in our purses or have a stash in the car. Heaven forbid we should go longer than three hours without food—or even worse, get hungry!

Over the years, new studies show that these theories are not true, and although they may work for a small percentage of people like bodybuilders or athletes, the average person does not need to snack throughout the day. Three meals, and in some cases even two larger meals, are sufficient for maintaining and achieving a healthy weight.

The result of the 'snacking' theory did not help people trying to lose weight; in fact, it had the opposite effect.

According to a new study, Americans eat roughly 570 calories more per day than they did in the 1970s. While supersize portions are partly to blame, steady snacking is the bigger culprit.

Before you get a snack, check your motivation. Ask yourself the following questions: Are you doing it out of habit? Do you really need a snack? Can you drink some water instead?

Here's the truth, and the research supporting it:

1. Eating smaller meals more often does not increase your metabolism. See the research here[6].

2. It's a myth that snacking is better for weight loss than eating three meals per day. Contrary to this belief, going for longer periods of time without food has been proven to have major health benefits such as diabetes prevention[7], decreased inflammation[8], and weight loss[9].

3. If snacking helps reduce your cravings and contributes to helping you eat less overall, then do it;

6   https://www.ncbi.nlm.nih.gov/pubmed/9155494
7   https://www.sciencedirect.com/science/article/pii/S193152441400200X
8   https://www.ncbi.nlm.nih.gov/pmc/articles/PMC3946160/
9   https://www.ncbi.nlm.nih.gov/pmc/articles/PMC3946160/

otherwise, it is not an effective weight-loss tool—in most cases, it has the opposite effect.

Action

Today, you're going to challenge yourself to eat only at breakfast, lunch and dinner—no snacking.

Reflect

1. If you do snack, calculate how many additional calories you consume each day in snacks. Be sure to pay attention to what a serving size is. Eg. One large apple may be two servings. Do they sabotage your efforts?

   _____

   _____

   _____

   _____

2. Why do you find yourself snacking? Is it boredom, loneliness, habit? Journal some of the reasons you snack.

   _____

   _____

   _____

   _____

3. What time of the day do you feel you need a snack? Is there something you can do instead?

   _____

   _____

   _____

   _____

4. What are some healthy alternatives to your favorite non-nutritious snack foods? Eg. air-popped corn vs chips. Soda water with juice vs. colas.

_____

_____

_____

_____

Prayer

"Dear Lord, snacking has always been part of my lifestyle so the thought of going without it scares me. What if I get too hungry in between meals? What if I end up bingeing because I got too hungry? What if my blood sugar falls too low or I get headaches or nauseated because I'm so hungry? So many questions, Lord. But even as I reflect on all of these thoughts right now, I realize that they are all based on fear. You continue to show me that I need to have more faith in You and less fear of what might or might not happen. So today, I bring another fear to You, Lord, and I lay it at Your feet. Help me to be mindful of my unnecessary snacking. Let me be mindful if I'm snacking out of habit, emotion, or fear. And remind me that I can turn to You and let go of this and any other way of being that does not serve me or glorify You. When I feel like I 'need a little something', remind me that You are enough. Remind me that my satisfaction comes from You and I don't need to hunger for anything other than You. In Your Name I pray. Amen!"

My Prayer

_____

_____

_____

_____

_____

_____

_____

_____

_____

_____

Additional Scriptures

"Their end is destruction, their god is their belly, and they glory in their shame, with minds set on earthly things."
~Philippians 3:19

"But the fruit of the Spirit is love, joy, peace, patience, kindness, goodness, faithfulness, gentleness, self-control; against such things there is no law." ~Galatians 5:22-23

"All things are lawful for me, but not all things are helpful. All things are lawful for me, but I will not be enslaved by anything." ~1 Corinthians 6:12

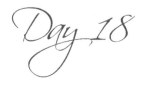

Listening to Your Body

Scripture Reflection

"I praise you because I am fearfully and wonderfully made;
your works are wonderful, I know that full well."
~Psalms 139:14

Devotion

It's hard to praise God when we don't believe we're fearfully and wonderfully made. The psalmist says, 'I know that full well''. Could you say the same? Can you, and do you, praise God for creating you so wonderfully? Or have you disconnected from its wonder, and therefore are not able to give God praise?

Unfortunately, many of us have disconnected from our bodies. We no longer look in the mirror because we don't like the reflection looking back at us, and we've paid attention to how our actions or lack of them impact our health. But when we truly believe that our bodies are God's temple and we have a responsibility to nourish them and take care of them, we will start to appreciate them as God does.

It's up to you to do your homework to understand your body and its unique needs, then feed it what it needs.

The best way to do this is to begin to pay attention and listen to your body. It's talking to you every day. So, what is it saying to you? And, more importantly, are you listening?

There are many ways in which your body speaks to you. Some of the obvious conversations are hunger, thirst, bathroom breaks, and tiredness. But what about skin rashes, headaches, indigestion, constipation, and even muscle cramps? These are all signals that something is not working right in your body's system. Your body not only communicates to the necessary nerves, cells, and hormones, but it communicates to you also. Learning to hear what your body is saying is not hard; it just requires your time and attention.

Food cravings, food sensitivities, bodyweight issues, gas and bloating, and abdominal discomfort are ways in which your body signals to you that your DIGESTIVE SYSTEM is compromised. Your digestive system includes your mouth, esophagus, stomach, intestines, rectum, and anus. They all play a part in breaking down food, digesting nutrients, and eliminating waste from our bodies. This system is largely affected by food choices and, you guessed it, stress.

The best place to start is by simply being aware of what's going on in your body. What is your body telling you right now? Is there pain anywhere? Are you sleepy? Do you feel anxious? Don't ignore the signals anymore. The headaches, poor sleeping habits, and food cravings are just your body's way of speaking to you. Like the check-engine light that comes on in your car to indicate that something is wrong, your body will often tell you when it needs your attention. It's time to be more attentive.

When you're tuned in to your body, you won't have to waste money on vitamins and potions that weren't meant for you. Sure, they may work for your friend, but that does not mean that they are the best thing for your body. My body needs a daily iron supplement because it does not produce enough, but that does not apply to everyone. Someone else's body may not produce another nutrient and amino acid that may be specific only to their unique body. Secondly, when you're eating a healthy diet, it will provide you with an adequate supply of vitamins and nutrients that you need. You may not even need to supplement.

When you're tuned in to your body, you won't have to waste countless hours on the treadmill or Stairmaster. Those machines might work for your friend, but your body might be telling you that it only needs a light walk or to be stretched.

When you're tuned in to your body, you can rid yourself of all the guilt and pressure of what you think you 'should' be doing. You won't have to force it or even guess what you need to do; your body will simply tell you. Imagine having that kind of freedom. Tightness in your shoulder? Perform some stretches. Feeling sluggish? Head outside for a walk and get some vitamin D, or drink some more water and see what difference it makes in how you feel.

Action

Today, with a journal on hand, listen to how your body is talking to you. Pay attention to signals of hunger, gas, bloating, energy levels, overeating, and mood.

- Why did you eat? Were you hungry?
- How did you feel after you ate? Were you satisfied? Sleepy? Did you crave something sweet?
- If you broke your boundaries, what were you craving?
- How did you feel when you went to sleep?
- How often is food on your mind? How much time, energy, or attention do you give to eating?
- How many hours do you go between meals?
- Are you drinking the appropriate amount of water for your body?

- What is the ideal meal that makes you feel the best? Why don't you eat more of it?
- How are your energy levels before and after eating?
- What foods is your body craving?

Reflect

1. What does it mean that we are fearfully and wonderfully made? Do you truly believe it?

   _____

   _____

   _____

   _____

2. How do you treat your body like it's fearfully and wonderfully made?

   _____

   _____

   _____

   _____

3. What do you think your body is telling you most of the time?

   _____

   _____

   _____

   _____

4. How can you speak to your body in a way that is in line with the Word of God?

   _____

   _____

   _____

Prayer

"Dear Lord, I thank You that I am fearfully and wonderfully made. It's amazing to know that I am created in Your image. What a privilege. Help me to tune into my body and remember this today as I eat. Holy Spirit, help me to be sensitive to what I feed my body and help me to only feed it foods that will strengthen and nourish it as You lead me away from foods that will harm it. I've disconnected from my body over the years, but now as I reconnect, help me to do so in a healthy way—in a way that glorifies You and brings praise to You. I lay aside every snare and stronghold that will keep me from understanding my body and keeping it in its rightful place. I control my body, it does not control me. Now I let go and rest in the truth that my body is Your temple. In Your Name I pray. Amen!"

My Prayer

_____

_____

_____

_____

_____

_____

_____

_____

_____

_____

Additional Scriptures

"This day I call the heavens and the earth as witnesses against you that I have set before you life and death, blessings and curses. Now choose life, so that you and your children may live and that you may love the Lord your God, listen to his voice, and hold fast to him." ~Deuteronomy 30:19–20

"For I know the plans I have for you," declares the Lord, "plans to prosper you and not to harm you, plans to give you hope and a future." ~Jeremiah 29:11

"And God said, Let us make man in our image, after our likeness: and let them have dominion over the fish of the sea, and over the fowl of the air, and over the cattle, and overall the earth, and over every creeping thing that creepeth upon the earth ..." ~Genesis 1:26–27

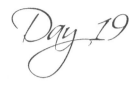

Food Addiction or Gluttony

Scripture Reflection

"You say, I am allowed to do anything—but not everything is good for you. And even though I am allowed to do anything, I must not become a slave to anything."
~1 Corinthians 6:12 (NLT)

Devotion

Part of this devotion is from one of our *Weight Loss, God's Way* members who shared her testimony about her uncle.

"Any of these sound familiar? This was my reality. When I came to terms with food addiction, I remember showing my husband all my hiding places for food. I was humiliated that I had allowed it to go so far.

- *Hiding junk food behind nutritious food so no one would find it*
- *Eating a salad in the presence of people then running home to eat high-fat, high-sugar, calorie-laden foods*
- *Going into the gas station to buy snacks at the same time you buy gas so it wouldn't show up on the receipt*
- *Having a secret stash of food in my bedside table, purse, desk drawers*
- *Eating to the point of physical discomfort or pain*

- *When going to the grocery store, you get cashback so you can go through the drive-thru and have no evidence in the bank account*

I've decided to come 'clean' as I thought about my uncle.

"God gave me free will and I will use it with food." This is what he said to me after one of his heart attacks. He struggled with diabetes and had multiple strokes and heart attacks. All of his health issues were due to his unhealthy diet. His doctor had warned him he needed to change his eating habits, but he refused to listen. He hid his snacks to eat when no one was around, just like I did. Like so many of us, he used his free will as an excuse to eat himself to his grave.

But when I stumbled across the scripture in 1 Corinthians 6:12 (NLT), I actually found it comforting. If this was a struggle that the disciples faced, why would I think I won't struggle with this, too? But the scripture was not meant to be used as a loop-hole, but as a reminder that we also need to exercise wisdom and common sense.

When my uncle passed, I was sad and mad at the same time. I was sad that I lost him. I was mad about what he had told me about his freewill with food. God gently nudged me one day and said that I have that same attitude. I just don't speak it out loud. I felt convicted immediately." ~ By Cynthia Bussey

The lines can be very blurry between food addictions, eating disorders, (spirit of) gluttony, or addictive foods. Coupled with that is our propensity to believe that our eating habits are out of our control. It's easier to blame a food addiction than it is to take responsibility for your habits, but even addicts need to take responsibility for the addiction if they are ever going to change. So let's get clear on some of the distinctions.

Food Addictions

Food addicts respond to food like a drug addict responds to drugs. The cause is likely the culmination of several factors including biological, psychological, or social reasons. As food increases the feeling of pleasure and reward, the addict needs more and more to feel better. Join a support group[10] that can help you overcome your food addictions.

Eating Disorders

These are more of a mental health disorder that has more to do with the behavior than the food itself. These require medical attention.

Addictive Foods

There are many foods on the market that are designed to make you eat more. They are known as hyper-palatable foods and their composition (sugar, fat, and salt) makes them easy to compulsively eat. These include foods like chips, french fries, chocolate, and ice cream. Avoid these foods altogether.

Spirit of Gluttony

The spirit of gluttony includes all of the conditions above. It is defined as an inordinate need to eat more than we desire. So if you just like the taste of food, and as a result overeat, you're still dealing with a spirit of gluttony. If you struggle with your weight for whatever reason, then it's important to acknowledge that you have a spirit of gluttony.

Regardless of which category you may find yourself in, treat gluttony as a sin and commit to stop overeating with the understanding that God must be an intricate part of your

---

10   https://www.foodaddicts.org/am-i-a-food-addict

recovery. In addition to prayer and knowing what God's Word says, here are a few other strategies to practice:

1. Admit that food is a stronghold for you and continually turn this journey over to God.

2. Have an accountability person you can be honest with and who will be strong enough to call you out when necessary.

3. Identify what trigger foods you struggle with and remove them from your home.

4. Stop hiding food or 'saving it for a special time'.

5. Without judgment, be ruthless and treat gluttony as a sin and repent.

Action

Repent today for your spirit of gluttony. Pour your heart out to God and let Him know your true desire to stop. Write out all the feelings, thoughts, and fears that come up and turn them all over to Him. Then thank Him for hearing and answering your prayers.

Reflect

1. When it comes to food, do your public and private life line up? In other words, do you eat differently in private when no one is looking?

   _____

   _____

   _____

2. Do you try to justify your food choices so that you can still have what you want?

_____

_____

_____

3. Do you judge what others are eating, but in secret you eat the things you know you shouldn't eat?

_____

_____

_____

Prayer

"Father God, thank You for the victory over our strongholds. I bind the spirit of gluttony that lives in me, in Your Name. Forgive me for eating the things that I know don't benefit the body You have given me. Forgive me, Lord, for choosing to ignore Your Word and the doctor's guidance in how I should eat. Thank You for loving me so much that You want to encourage me to change. Continue to convict me in areas that need to be changed. Break the strongholds of addiction, in Jesus' Name. Amen."

My Prayer

_____

_____

_____

_____

_____

_____

_____

Additional Scriptures

*"I don't really understand myself, for I want to do what is
right, but I don't do it. Instead, I do what I hate."*
~Romans 7:15 (NLT)

*"The temptations in your life are no different from what
others experience. And God is faithful. He will not allow the
temptation to be more than you can stand. When you are
tempted, he will show you a way out so that you can endure.
14 So, my dear friends, flee from the worship of idols."*
~1 Corinthians 10:13 (NLT)

*"They are headed for destruction. Their god is their appetite,
they brag about shameful things, and they think only about
this life here on earth." ~Philippians 3:19 (NLT)*

*"So whether you eat or drink, or whatever you do, do it all for
the glory of God." ~1 Corinthians 10:31 (NLT)*

*"Look, this was the iniquity of your sister Sodom: She and
her daughter had pride, fullness of food, and abundance of
idleness; neither did she strengthen the hand of the poor and
needy. And they were haughty and committed abomination
before Me; therefore I took them away as I saw fit."*
~Ezekiel 16:49-50

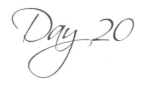

Overcoming Food Temptations

Scripture Reflection

> *"Just before His arrest, Jesus was in the Garden of Gethsemane, and He said to His disciples, 'Watch and pray so that you will not fall into temptation. The spirit is willing, but the flesh is weak.'" ~Matthew 26:41*

Devotion

Ever get frustrated at how often you give in to your cravings and temptations?

This is a good time to remember that in our flesh, we will never be able to consistently resist temptations—our flesh is just too weak. The Bible says, "The spirit is willing, but the flesh is weak."

This Scripture is taken from the gospel of Matthew. The conversation takes place right after the Last Supper. Judas had left the dinner to orchestrate the betrayal of Jesus and now we find Jesus agonizing in the Garden of Gethsemane. He is talking to the disciples (specifically Peter) and is warning him about the weakness of his physical body as he grows sleepy, and Jesus reminds him how easily his body will give in to temptations.

If we apply this scripture in Matthew 26:41 to the context of your weight-loss journey, it means that you may really want to eat well but you're just not able to muster up the energy/ discipline/motivation or drive to actually do it.

The 'flesh' Jesus referred to in the Scripture above is our physical body with its appetites, desires, and weaknesses, always looking for the easy way out. Your flesh easily gives in to temptation. Remember that reptile brain and that monkey brain we keep talking about? Well here it is again! Your flesh will always overpower your spirit if you don't watch and pray as Jesus instructed the disciples to do, as was the case with the disciples.

How does Jesus instruct us? To WATCH AND PRAY!

Watch

You will give in to temptation when you're not 'standing on guard'.

You need to guard your minds and your emotions like a hen taking care of her chicks. If you let anything into your mind it will wear down your spirit, so be mindful of the friends who are always inviting you out to the fast food restaurants, watching the enticing food channels, or even perusing all the food photos on Pinterest. Are you spending time with people who bring you down or build you up—'leaners' or 'lifters'?

- Do you continue to visit fast-food restaurants and drive-thrus and hope you won't be tempted?
- Do you continue to live outside of your boundaries?

These will all continue to wear you down.

Also pay attention to your emotions because the enemy will 'attack' when your resistance is low. That's why we use the acronym H.A.L.T. Don't allow yourself to get too 'Hungry, Angry, Lonely, or Tired'.

- If you're too stressed, your flesh will grow weak.
- If you're too emotional about a situation, your flesh will grow weak.
- If you're sleep-deprived, your flesh will grow weak.
- If you're not properly hydrated or fueled with nutritious foods, your flesh will grow weak.

Your flesh will be more willing when it is well-rested, well-fed both physically and spiritually, and feeling at peace. That's when your resistance will be strongest.

Pray

Jesus prepared the disciples by telling them to pray.

The struggle was real for Jesus, too! He just finished practicing this same principle with the disciples. We learn in the earlier verses that His flesh was failing Him, so He prayed to God to be strengthened. The Bible says, *"And after going a little farther, He fell face-down and prayed, saying, 'My Father, if it is possible [that is, consistent with Your will], let this cup pass from Me; yet not as I will, but as You will'"* (Matthew 26:39). The same God who strengthened Jesus when He prayed to Him is the same God who will strengthen you during your periods of weakness, trials, and temptations.

Action

As you go about your day today, in addition to your action step practice watching and praying before you eat anything.

Reflect

1. What keeps you from watching and praying about your eating boundaries? Turn it over to God right now in prayer.

   _____

   _____

   _____

   _____

2. What do you need to be most watchful of? Journal it.

   _____

   _____

   _____

   _____

3. Write out a prayer to God, letting Him know your desire to stay within your healthy eating boundaries.

   _____

   _____

   _____

   _____

Prayer

"Dear Lord, giving in to my temptations is one of the most frustrating parts of my journey. I start the day feeling strong and encouraged, but as the day goes by I just get weaker and weaker until I feel so defeated. Then I wake up the next day and start the same cycle over and over again. I'm grateful that I am learning how to identify why I keep repeating this pattern. I'm also glad that I'm learning that I am not powerless—I am not a victim. But I am also no match for my cravings, and that's why

I must pray. I must come to You every time and I must stand on guard so that You will fight my battles for me. So I take a deep breath, I let go of all the anxiety I have around my fears of never overcoming my temptations. I watch, I pray, and I trust that You will help me. You will strengthen me. You will satisfy my hunger and cravings. Thank You, Lord. In Your Name I pray. Amen."

My Prayer

_____

_____

_____

_____

_____

_____

_____

_____

Additional Scriptures

"No temptation has overtaken you except what is common to mankind. And God is faithful; he will not let you be tempted beyond what you can bear. But when you are tempted, he will also provide a way out so that you can endure it."
~1 Corinthians 10:13

"The prudent see danger and take refuge, but the simple keep going and pay the penalty." ~Proverbs 22:3

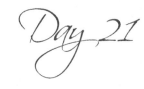
Day 21

Week 3 Summary

Scripture Reflection

"Give thanks to the LORD, for he is good; his love endures forever." ~Psalms 107:1

Congratulations on completing week 3!

As we wrap up this week, review what you have learned.

1. Recap

What are you learning about healthy eating so far?

2. Reflect

Journal what the Holy Spirit is showing you so far. How many days did you practice your action step?

3. Pray

Commit your week to the Lord. Thank Him for bringing you through the past week and preparing you for the final week.

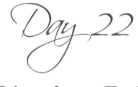

Staying Full

Scripture Reflection

"For he satisfies the thirsty and fills the hungry with good things." ~Psalms 107:9

Devotion

Confession time here ... I've been known to drive for miles and miles (kilometers here in Canada) before putting gas in the car. When that 'low fuel' light came on, I often ignored it for at least a couple of days. It became like a game of 'let's see how far I can go before I run out of gas'. What an overrated game when you think about it. Aside from a small adrenaline rush, feeling like I survived another trip, letting the car run on fumes is always a bad plan.

Our human bodies operate in a similar fashion. Sadly, waiting to fill the tank until I'm running on fumes is an all too familiar pattern in my life, too. My emotions can have a big impact on what I eat. I don't often recognize when I'm doing it but it shows up as dissatisfaction, apathy, and wanting to abandon my goals. I feel tired, have no energy, and start looking for shortcuts in everything I do. Then I keep doing things to try to make myself feel better, but nothing works. You know that feeling where no matter what you eat you just can't get full? It happens to me spiritually as well as physically.

So what's the 'trick' to stop running on empty both emotionally and spiritually? Stay FULL! As much as this applies to food, I'm talking about staying full of the Word of God.

When we're full, we don't have to push the limits to see how long we can run on empty. God's Word will provide us with so much encouragement and peace that we won't feel the need to push past our limits.

When we're spiritually full, we don't have to keep going through the emotional highs and lows that accompany running on fumes.

As I did a bit of research on car maintenance, I learned that maintaining a full tank of gas is better for the engine than waiting for the gas light to come on. It prevents fuel pump failure and prevents dirt from getting trapped in the fuel tank. Wow!

Staying with this analogy, I'm so tired of letting 'dirt' get trapped in my mind. My stinkin' thinkin' will wreak havoc in my mind if it stays too long. I want peace. I want freedom. I want joy in the Lord. All of that is available when I (we) remain in God's Word and seek satisfaction and fulfillment from Him alone.

Action

Today, you're going to experience what it feels like to stay full of the Word of God. Practice praying ceaselessly. Pray as soon as you wake up, give God thanks for everything you do. Pray as you move from one room to the next and one activity to the next. Pray before you talk to anyone and pray for anyone that crosses your path. And of course pray before you eat and after you eat. Journal your experience.

Reflect

1. What are some indications that you're running on low fuel both physically and spiritually?

_____

_____

_____

2. Have you ever confused spiritual hunger with physical hunger? How can you tell the difference?

_____

_____

_____

3. What happens when you try to fill spiritual hunger with food?

_____

_____

_____

4. How does being in the Word refuel you?

_____

_____

_____

Worship and Prayer

"Lord, I thank You that you fill me completely with joy and peace. I trust You to meet all of my needs—emotionally and spiritually. I will continue to feast on Your words so that I will never allow myself to run on empty and that I will never operate in excess either. You give me just what I need. I will hide Your Word in my heart; it is like a lamp that guides me in the darkness. When I'm feeling stuck, it's Your Word that will see me through. Although it's never my intention, the next time I'm running on fumes, let me run to You for nourishment instead of seeking things that don't satisfy me. In Your Holy and precious Name I pray. Amen."

My Prayer

_____

_____

_____

_____

_____

_____

_____

_____

_____

Additional Scriptures

"How sweet are your words to my taste, sweeter than honey to my mouth!" ~Psalms 119:103

"As the deer pants for the water brooks, So my soul pants for You, O God." ~Psalms 42:1

"For it was I, the Lord your God, who rescued you from the land of Egypt. Open your mouth wide, and I will FILL IT with good things." ~Psalms 81:10

"He FILLS my life with good things. My youth is renewed like the eagle's!" ~Psalms 103:5

"For he satisfies the thirsty and FILLS the hungry with good things." ~Psalms 107:9

"Don't be drunk with wine, because that will ruin your life. Instead, be FILLED with the Holy Spirit." ~Ephesians 5:18

"When your words came, I ate them; they were my joy and my heart's delight, for I bear your name, Lord God Almighty." ~Jeremiah 15:16

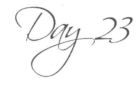

My Food is My Food

Scripture Reflection

"Please test your servants for ten days. Let us be given only vegetables to eat and water to drink. Then compare our appearances with those of the young men who are eating the royal food, and deal with your servants according to what you see." ~Daniel 1:12‑13

Devotion

Doesn't it feel like life isn't fair sometimes? Gorgeous Sherry can eat whatever she wants and never gain a pound, and you only have to look at food and you're up five pounds. It feels unfair, doesn't it? And we can probably find many other instances in life where we don't feel like things are fair. Mary has the perfect husband and yours is just ... meh. Laura has this amazing hair that always looks like she just walked out of a salon; meanwhile, your best hair day looks like you stuck your finger in a light socket.

Truth is, it is not up to us to judge what is fair and what is not fair. God calls us to walk our own path. He has made us all different. We need to accept this and stop comparing ourselves to others and focus on ourselves.

As difficult and as painful as it might be to face, feeling a sense of unfairness about what we can or cannot eat comes from a spirit of entitlement (I deserve this treatment because …), a spirit of jealousy (I want what they have …), or a spirit of control (I want what I want …).

As we learn to walk in the Spirit, we will learn to fix our eyes above and not on how we think things should be. We will learn to let go of our expectations and believe and trust God.

Facts:

- We can't eat the way we did when we were teenagers.
- If we go on a diet with our husbands, they will probably drop weight faster than us.
- We can't eat what other people eat.

Accept these truths and move on.

Let your food be your food and stop feeling bad that you can't eat cake. There are many things that you can enjoy. God has given you a variety and He has given them to you for your own health and safety. He knows what's best for you and what foods will allow your body to thrive.

Daniel could have given in to the feast. After all, he was in the king's palace. He was in a foreign land where no one would have been the wiser. He probably could smell the aroma of all the delectable foods and was probably hungry from living on vegetables and water. But his commitment was to God. Even under duress or pressure, he wanted God to be glorified. We often focus so much on what others will think, we feel we should be entitled because 'you don't know the rough week I had' or we feel that life is not fair.

Action

Today, make a list of all 'Your Foods',' then post it on your fridge or somewhere that you can see it often. Include all the foods you enjoy eating, that taste good, and satisfy you. Make it a point to enjoy those foods today and as often as you can.

Reflect

1. What foods allow you to perform at your best— energizing and revitalizing you?

   _____

   _____

   _____

2. Why did Daniel refuse to eat the king's food?

   _____

   _____

   _____

3. How was he able to maintain his strength and energy despite the 'meager' diet?

   _____

   _____

   _____

4. Do you have any resentment about what you can and cannot eat? Turn it over to God in prayer today.

   _____

   _____

   _____

Prayer

"Dear Lord, I thank You for providing me with foods that nourish my body. They are designed specifically for my unique needs and I'm so grateful for that. You have created me so uniquely, my body is like no other. Help me to be grateful for everything that I have instead of focusing on what I can't eat, do, or be. Help me to accept all that I am and all that I am not. Give me a spirit of gratitude and thankfulness and mature me so that there is no jealousy, envy, entitlement, or need to control. I walk with a spirit of contentment. Satisfy me with the foods that are within my boundaries and turn my eyes away from all other foods. Make me be the woman who accepts what You have for me and let me celebrate it by giving You glory. In Your Name I pray. Amen!"

My Prayer

_____

_____

_____

_____

_____

_____

_____

_____

_____

_____

_____

Additional Scriptures

"And he humbled thee, and suffered thee to hunger, and fed thee with manna, which thou knewest not, neither did thy fathers know; that he might make thee know that man doth not live by bread only, but by every word that proceedeth out of the mouth of the LORD doth man live." ~Deuteronomy 8:3

"The people asked, and he brought quails, and satisfied them with the bread of heaven." ~Psalms 105:40

"And the Lord will guide you continually and satisfy your desire in scorched places and make your bones strong; and you shall be like a watered garden, like a spring of water, whose waters do not fail." ~Isaiah 58:11.

"And if the spirit of jealousy comes over him and he is jealous of his wife who has defiled herself, or if the spirit of jealousy comes over him and he is jealous of his wife, though she has not defiled herself." ~Numbers 5:14

I Deserve a Treat

Scripture Reflection

"Have this mind among yourselves, which is yours in Christ Jesus, who, though he was in the form of God, did not count equality with God a thing to be grasped, but emptied himself, by taking the form of a servant, being born in the likeness of men. And being found in human form, he humbled himself by becoming obedient to the point of death, even death on a cross." ~Philippians 2:5-8

Devotion

We only need to turn on the TV to get bombarded with an onslaught of messages telling us what we deserve:

- We deserve to live the 'good' life.
- We deserve to have it all.
- We deserve to drink this particular beer and drive this type of car.

It's so easy to get caught up in the world's system of what is fair and what is not. But as Christian women, we don't have to give in to the world's systems—especially when God has provided us with an alternative to the world's flawed system.

- The world says, "Work really hard and you will make it to the top."

God says *"Humble yourselves, therefore, under God's mighty hand, that he may lift you up in due time." ~1 Peter 5:6 NLT*

- The world says, "That person has been mean to you and does not deserve your friendship."

God says, *"But I tell you, love your enemies and pray for those who persecute you." ~Matthew 5:44*

- The world says, "You've had a tough week, so you deserve a treat."

God says, *"Whoever wants to be my disciple must deny themselves and take up their cross and follow me." ~Matthew 16:24*

The world's ways are not our ways (Isaiah 55:8-9). We know that intuitively because we keep trying and it keeps getting us into trouble. God's ways provide freedom. He knows what's best for us because He knows the entire picture. Our perspective is like a grain of sand compared to His.

Sister, you have been delivered from the world's system of fairness and entitlement. You no longer have to fight to get what is owed to you. God is fair and perfectly righteous in His treatment of his sons and daughters.

To overcome your entitlement issues, live your life in obedience to God's Word and experience the satisfaction that comes from trusting that God is fair, righteous, and just.

Living a life of contentment without telling ourselves what we deserve requires the perspective and courage to choose God's ways over what feels most deserving at the time. Choose to base fairness and entitlement in God's economy and not the world's. The Holy Spirit will help you to understand what is fair and what is not. Choose to let go of all feelings of entitlement, and experience the satisfaction that comes from living your life within the safety and security of the boundaries that the Lord has set for you.

Action

For today, pay attention to your entitlement or fairness (or lack of fairness) thinking. Journal them and then use God's Word to confront your beliefs. How does God's Word change your perspective on what you deserve?

Reflect

1. What do you do that makes you feel worthy and deserving of a treat?

    _____

    _____

    _____

    _____

2. How does Philippians 2:5-8 teach us that humility is important to help us overcome our sense of entitlement?

    _____

    _____

    _____

    _____

3. How is God's standard for fairness different from the world's standards?

    _____

    _____

    _____

    _____

4. What will you do the next time you feel that you deserve a treat or something outside your boundaries?

_____

_____

_____

Prayer

"Heavenly Father, I thank You for always saving me from myself. Please forgive my propensity to think that I know what I deserve or what's best for me. I've been wrong every single time. I can't see the whole picture so I can't possibly know what's best for me, but You do. Help me to trust you. You have never led me astray, Daddy. It's not about what I deserve but about what You deserve, and You deserve all the glory, all the honor, and all the praise! In Jesus' Name, Amen."

My Prayer

_____

_____

_____

_____

_____

_____

_____

_____

_____

_____

Additional Scriptures

"As obedient children, do not be conformed to the former lusts which were yours in your ignorance, but like the Holy One who called you, be holy yourselves also in all your behavior; because it is written, 'You shall be holy, for I am holy.'" ~1 Peter 1:14-16

"Not that I speak from want, for I have learned to be content in whatever circumstances I am." ~Philippians 4:11

"God opposes the proud, but gives grace to the humble." ~James 4:6

"He also told this parable to some who trusted in themselves that they were righteous, and treated others with contempt: 10 'Two men went up into the temple to pray, one a Pharisee and the other a tax collector. The Pharisee, standing by himself, prayed thus: 'God, I thank you that I am not like other men, extortioners, unjust, adulterers, or even like this tax collector. I fast twice a week; I give tithes of all that I get.' But the tax collector, standing far off, would not even lift up his eyes to heaven, but beat his breast, saying, 'God, be merciful to me, a sinner!' I tell you, this man went down to his house justified, rather than the other. For everyone who exalts himself will be humbled, but the one who humbles himself will be exalted." ~Luke 18:9-14

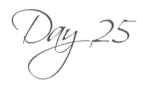

Food Lies

Scripture Reflection

"Then you will know the truth, and the truth will set you free." ~John 8:32

Devotion

In her book, *Taste for Truth,* Barb Raveling states that the strongholds we experience around our health are based on lies. Could it be that simple? Okay, ask yourself these questions:

- Do you really believe that just one bite won't hurt? Really?
- Do you really believe that a particular food will make you feel better?
- Do you really not have the time to prepare nutritious foods?
- Are you really powerless against your food addiction?
- Will you really start your diet tomorrow?
- Did you really have no choice in the matter?
- Do you really need to have dessert after a meal?
- Do you really believe that you can't go without a meal?

It's time to tell yourself the truth. It's time to get real and hold yourself accountable for the self-defeating thoughts that hold you back. It's time to hold yourself accountable for the conscious lies that you tell yourself as you pray that the subconscious lies will be brought to the surface.

Very few of us would ever call ourselves liars. In fact, if we were challenged on some of the things we say, many of us would bet some cold hard cash that we're telling the truth. Yet here's the thing—RESULTS NEVER LIE! If you're not getting the results that you've been seeking, then there are some truths that you have not been telling yourself.

Reasons we don't tell ourselves the truth

There are many reasons we lie to ourselves:

1. We've believed the lies for so long that it's become our truth.
2. We did not know it was a lie.
3. We have a low standard for the truth.
4. It's less painful to lie than to face the truth.
5. The enemy has deceived us.

Despite why we do it, commit to being 100% truthful with yourself. Start by doing this:

1. Don't trust yourself!

The Bible says, *"The heart is deceitful above all things and beyond cure. Who can understand it?"* ~Jeremiah 17:9

Regardless of what you tell yourself in the heat of the moment, if you have not been successful in the past do not trust what your mind is telling you at the moment. Do what you know to do and do not trust yourself to make the right decisions for yourself when it comes to your health.

Get present to your thoughts and your speech and boldly tell yourself that it is a lie. It is not true that you will only have one bite. Remind yourself that past history dictates that it is not possible to have one bite.

2. Replace every lie with the truth.

As long as we allow lies to run roughshod in our minds, we will continue to struggle with our weight and our health. We must treat these lies like a contagious, infectious disease that will slowly destroy every cell in our body if we allow it to.

The Bible is clear on how we are to eradicate lies from our minds and our lives. We are to *"bring every thought into captivity to the obedience of Christ." ~2 Corinthians 10:5b*

3. Face the truth and trust that God will cover you (Psalm 91:4).

God will only cover what you're willing to uncover. This means that God will give you grace and strength in those areas that you feel are too difficult, too ugly, or too painful to face or even to share with Him. Lying to yourself ties God's hands, because you're choosing to control the situation by keeping the truth from yourself and from God. Although God already knows, He needs you to see the truth for yourself in order for transformation to take place. As painful as it sounds, you're choosing your truth over God's truth.

When you find yourself wanting to hide because you want to break your boundaries, admit to God that you're unable to do things on your own. You can't handle the truth, but believe without a shadow of a doubt that God can.

4. Get accountability.

The final tool in our arsenal for eradicating lies in our lives is to be accountable to others. We simply cannot trust ourselves to tell ourselves the truth, so that's why accountability is important. Because we've believed the lies for so long that they've become our truth, because we may have a low standard for truth, and because we may not recognize the lies that we tell ourselves, we need to be accountable to others.

Proverbs 27:17 teaches us that, *"As iron sharpens iron, so a man sharpens the countenance of his friend."*

We were called to bear each other's burdens. Commit to sharing your journey each day, and commit to lovingly challenge others when you notice that they are not telling themselves the truth.

Action

Write out all the 'lies' you tell yourself when you don't practise your action step that you committed to. What is the truth found in God's Word that you will use to replace the lie?

Reflect

1. Write out three to four scriptures that you will declare when you notice you lying to yourself.

    _____

    _____

    _____

    _____

2. Who will you be accountable to so you do not continue lying to yourself?

    _____

    _____

    _____

    _____

3. What truth(s) about your health journey are you
    unwilling to face and need the Lord's strength?

    _____

    _____

    _____

    _____

4. Share one area of your weight-loss journey that
    you've been continually lying to yourself about.
    Do you keep telling yourself that you can do it on
    your own? Or that you have eaten certain foods in
    moderation? What is the truth about the situation?
    Get clear and honest about the real truth and spend
    some time journaling about it.

    _____

    _____

    _____

    _____

Worship and Prayer

"Dear Lord, You know my heart completely; I cannot lie to You
even if I tried! Search me and bring the areas where I am lying
to myself to light. Take that darkness and make it as plain as
day. I honor You in all areas of my life and I am a witness to all
You are doing in me. Thank You for Your Word and the promises
contained in them. I speak them into my life and replace my lies
with Your truth! In Jesus' Name I pray. Amen!"

My Prayer

_____

_____

_____

_____

_____

_____

_____

_____

_____

_____

Additional Scriptures

"The heart is deceitful above all things and beyond cure. Who can understand it?" ~Jeremiah 17:9

"Do not conform to the pattern of this world, but be transformed by the renewing of your mind." ~Romans 12:2

"We are to "bring every thought into captivity to the obedience of Christ." ~2 Corinthians 10:5

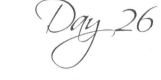

Grateful Eating

Scripture Reflection

"For everything created by God is good, and nothing is to be rejected if it is received with thanksgiving, for it is made holy by the word of God and prayer." ~1 Timothy 4:4-5

Devotion

To this day, I can still recite the same prayer we said every Sunday before dinner during my childhood years. I don't remember saying it before any other meal, but I distinctly remember that it had to be said for our special Sunday dinner. I found it odd that we needed to bless the food.

I remember a similar feeling as an adult. I often felt guilty blessing my McDonald's meal or some other highly non-nutritious meal. Maybe I felt like the prayer would somehow magically allow the food to provide nourishment for my body.

Both as a child and an adult, I never had a good understanding of why we needed to bless our food. As I studied my Bible, I learned that there is nowhere in the Bible where they actually blessed their meals. So why do we do it?

What the Bible tells us is that they gave thanks to God for their food. That's why we pray before we eat. All the prayers surrounding food was to express gratitude and thanks to God who provided for all their needs. By blessing God and thanking

Him for our food, it will help us to focus on God and to thank Him in every area of our lives.

If we're not mindful, mealtime prayers can become a meaningless ritual that we may not even give much thought to—especially if we say the same thing each time.

Here are some ways that we can practice gratitude for our food.

Treat every meal as a miracle.

When you think about what it took to get the food to the table, about what happens to the food when it enters your body, how it engages all five of our senses and how it's converted to energy, it's amazing that we no longer find this experience truly awe-inspiring. Treat every meal as the miracle that it truly is.

Pray with intentionality and thanksgiving.

We do not pray so that God will bless our food. Our food is no more or less blessed if we pray, but it allows us to take the time and thank God for all that He provides for us. It does not make us any more or less Christian. It's an opportunity to pause and think about God's goodness.

Don't fall into a rut.

If you're used to saying the same old boring prayers day in and day out, it's probably time for a change. Each time you sit down to a meal, think of a fresh new way to thank God for your meal. Identify one or two different things to thank God for. Get creative and keep your prayers fun and fresh.

Action

Pray before all your meals today, being intentional to change up your routine prayers. Pray differently today as you thank God in a way that you've never thanked Him before.

Reflect

1. How can your mealtime prayers change your perspective on what and how you eat?

    _____

    _____

    _____

2. Write out a prayer of thanksgiving to God for the food He has provided you.

    _____

    _____

    _____

3. As you eat a meal today, take some time and engage all of your senses. Pay attention to the smells, the texture of the food, the taste, the crunch, and give God thanks for it all. Thank him for your tastebuds, your sight, your sense of smell, and for the ability to experience them all.

    _____

    _____

    _____

Prayer

"Lord, I'm in awe at how You gave us food to delight our senses, to energize us, to nourish us, to strengthen our bodies, and to sustain us. When I think about the digestive process, how food enters and leaves our bodies, it's truly mind-boggling. Let me never ever take it for granted. Help me to eat slowly and see my food as the miracle that it truly is. Let me think of You and give You thanks, praise, and glory every time I eat. I truly thank You for the gift of food. Let me never take it for granted, let me never abuse it, and let me never use it as anything other than what You intended it for. Thank You again for giving me the miracle of food. In Your Name I pray. Amen!"

My Prayer

_____

_____

_____

_____

_____

_____

_____

_____

_____

_____

Additional Scriptures

"He gave thanks and broke the loaves." ~Matthew 14:19

"Whatever you do in word or deed, do everything in the name of the Lord Jesus, giving thanks to God the Father through Him." ~Colossians 3:17

"And when he had said these things, he took bread, and giving thanks to God in the presence of all he broke it and began to eat." ~Acts 27:35

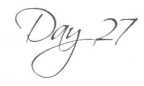

I've Got Food on My Mind

Scripture Reflection

"We demolish arguments and every pretension that sets itself up against the knowledge of God, and we take captive every thought to make it obedient to Christ." ~2 Corinthians 10:5

Devotion

Confession time. I used to think about food all the time. The second I opened my eyes, I thought about what I would eat for breakfast.

I would write out shopping lists and would indulge in what is now known as 'food porn'—salivating about all the foods I would eat and all the new recipes I would try. But it was okay because I always ate healthfully—until I didn't.

I could hold it together for a few weeks or even months, then I would 'lose it' and binge for weeks on end. I never made the connection between all of the mental thoughts, all the internet surfing, and all the obsessing I did about food.

About 15 years ago, I was involved in a heartbreaking relationship where the man I loved up and married another woman. I was devastated. What made matters worse was that we still attended the same church. A trusted friend of mine counseled me to throw out all of the photos I had of him, stop rereading his texts, stop thinking about all the good times we had together, and when

I saw him at church to walk in another direction so I did not have to breathe in his cologne and get sucked back into the sad saga again. *"I can't"*, I would tell her. *"I just can't stop thinking about him. You don't know what it's like."* Obviously, this was an unhealthy romance that would not have ended well.

It's the same with food. Do you have an unhealthy romance with food? Thinking about it all the time, walking past the bakery counter in the grocery store, is a bad plan.

Why put yourself in that situation? There is nothing noble about putting yourself in harm's way and then trying to resist. That's not noble, that's just unwise.

Chances are, food has taken up more brain space than you care to admit. Your monkey has been leading you around, making you feel like you can't stop, but the Bible tells us that we are to take every thought captive and make it obedient to Christ. God would never tell us to do the impossible. As you notice your mind starting to obsess about food, as you get drawn into 'food porn' on Pinterest and you linger too long in the dessert aisle at the grocery store, remember that there is nothing noble in trying to resist temptation. You do not need to look at tempting foods to try to prove to yourself how strong your will is. It's wiser to not look at the food at all. Do not give the devil a foothold by allowing the thoughts to come into your mind. Stop it before it takes root. You can do it in the strength of the Lord.

As we wrap up this devotional and challenge, I pray that you have recognized that healthful eating is as much a mental, emotional, and spiritual battle as it is a physical one, and I pray that you are now equipped with spiritual weapons and mental disciplines that you will continue to practise to win so you can nurture your health.

The goal of this devotional and challenge is two-fold.

1. To focus on one action step for almost one month by fully submitting it to the Lord.

2. To shine the light on areas of your healthful eating for at least one day, but now it's up to you to select the lessons that are most impactful for you and practice them day-in and day-out.

Action

Pay attention to how often you think about food in unhealthy ways throughout the day. It may be passing by a Starbucks, going to the cupboard even though you're not hungry, and eating a snack just because you're watching TV. Just for today, offer up a prayer, declaration, or confession every time you notice yourself thinking about food at inappropriate times. This is a tool that you will continue to use forever.

Reflect

1. How do you put yourself in compromising situations that make it difficult to maintain your boundaries?

    _____

    _____

    _____

    _____

2. When do you find yourself thinking or obsessing about food? When you're tired? Frustrated? Lonely? What can you do instead?

    _____

    _____

    _____

    _____

3. ACCEPT that the thought has come into your mind without judgment. ACKNOWLEDGE that it was because you're feeling stressed, or whatever the circumstance was, and stand in the truth that God is bigger than all your cravings. He will sustain you and give you what you need.

_____

_____

_____

_____

Prayer

"Dear Lord, thank You for equipping me with everything I need to take my thoughts captive. I've got to admit that controlling my thoughts feels like herding cats. It doesn't seem possible, because my thoughts consume and overpower me often. But, I stand on Your Word and if Your Word says that I can take every thought captive, then I believe You. Every time my mind starts to wander to food or other thoughts that do not serve me, let me think of You instead. I choose to think about those things that are "true, noble, right, pure, lovely, and admirable." I thank You that I have Your mind. In Your Name I pray. Amen!"

My Prayer

_____

_____

_____

_____

_____

Additional Scriptures

"Fix your gaze directly before you. Make level paths for your feet and take only ways that are firm. Do not swerve to the right or the left; keep your foot from evil." ~Proverbs 4:24-31

"But we have the mind of Christ." ~1 Corinthians 2:16

"Fix your thoughts on Jesus." ~Hebrews 3:1

Finally, brothers and sisters, whatever is true, whatever is noble, whatever is right, whatever is pure, whatever is lovely, whatever is admirable—if anything is excellent or praiseworthy—think about such things." ~Philippians 4:8

" ... and do not give the devil a foothold." ~Ephesians 4:27

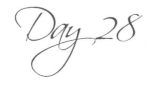

Putting it all Together

Scripture Reflection

"Whatever you have learned or received or heard from me, or seen in me—put it into practice. And the God of peace will be with you." ~Phil 4:9

Congratulations! You did it! You have begun to rewire your brain, realign your spirit, and retrain your taste buds to crave nutritious foods. You're well on your way to making changes that will serve you for the rest of your life.

You have developed a better understanding of how to invite God into this highly emotional, sometimes overwhelming, area of your life. You may have started this journey asking the question "What to eat?", which only kept you feeling frustrated and defeated.

Instead of asking yourself 'what to eat?' I hope that you will continue to ask yourself, *'Why aren't I eating the foods I know are healthful for me?'* And I pray that your query will always lead you back to Christ as He continues to satisfy your every spiritual hunger.

I pray that you have discovered that the answer to healthful eating lies in your willingness to submit this journey to God; that you've discovered that healthful eating is a lifestyle choice not to be entered in with the intention to just make changes to a few behaviours. God is looking for a heart change in you. And my last prayer for you is that you now see that healthful eating is as much about what's eating you as it is what you eat. It's as much about what you're craving spiritually as it is about your physical cravings for actual food.

Each day, I challenged you to examine one area of your healthful eating journey and consciously turn it over to God. It may have been your snacking, your water consumption, your lack of planning, or your spirit of gluttony. Whatever it is, I hope that you can now see that it's safe to turn it over to God and allow Him to help you. Like me, you've suffered in silence too long and the pain has been too great. You're now equipped with the freedom and peace that comes with healthful eating, God's way.

Reflect

Which of the lessons had the biggest impact on you? Read them again. Which ones had the Holy Spirit been speaking to you about for a while and perhaps this was just confirmation? Which lessons, when implemented, will have the greatest impact on your health and your weight? Start there!

Can you move the needle just slightly? Focus on one habit, surrender it to God, then rinse and repeat. You'll probably need to refer to some of these chapters again and again—perfect! Just like we go to church each week to keep our minds focused, you will also need to keep rehearsing these principles.

Remember, you got this—with the Lord as your strength.

Thank you for the opportunity of allowing me to share my perspective with you. Be blessed!

Closing Prayer

"Lord, I thank You for caring about every single detail of my life, including what I eat. Thank You for taking the time to explore my heart and show me the things in me that I'm unable to see with my own natural eyes. My spiritual eyes are open and I can see so much clearer how I've been sabotaging myself and eating my way through my challenges and trials instead of running to You. I have discovered so much and I'm trusting Your Holy Spirit to keep me mindful of these new revelations and to help me to keep putting into practice all of the new truths, habits, and new mindsets that I have learned. Every time I eat, I will offer up my food as a sacrifice to You. In Jesus' Name, Amen."

Just for Today

Each day you were introduced to a new healthful eating habit to practise that I believe when practised will help you to overcome some of the challenges you have with eating healthy. There may have been one, two, or even more that may have resonated with you and you may want to incorporate them into your eating plan more consistently. Here is a list of all of the daily action steps that you practised. Select one or more of them.

1. Getting Started. Track your daily consumption using a tracking app such as Myfitnesspal.com

2. Allow God to Search you. Read Psalms 139:23-34. Then read it again and ask God to search your heart and your mind to show you your anxious thoughts as they relate to your relationship with food.

3. Getting Clear on your Goal. Write out your health goal, getting clear on what you really want. Then pray and ask the Lord to show you a picture of what a healthy diet looks like for you.

4. Walking in the Spirit. Practice one of the spiritual disciplines when you notice your monkey brain

wanting to sabotage your actions (specifically the one you committed to on day one).

5. Managing Hunger. Experience what it feels like to be physically hungry. Write down what you're feeling physically, mentally, and even emotionally. Notice if it's physical hunger or brain hunger, and journal where in your body you're experiencing the feelings.

6. Planning for Success. Plan out all the steps involved in order to automate your action step so that it becomes a habit.

7. Understanding Macronutrients. Calculate your daily caloric needs if you don't already know it, and compare it to your current caloric consumption.

8. Meal Planning. Plan out your meal for an entire day.

9. Increasing Your Water consumption. Drink your required amount of water.

10. Practising Fasting. Practice the discipline of fasting from 6:00 A.M. to 6:00 P.M. (Note: if you have any health considerations, consult a medical practitioner on if this is appropriate for you and adjust accordingly.)

11. Feeling Your Feelings and Feeding Your Hunger. Track everything you eat then note either an "H" for hungry or "E" for emotional beside everything you eat.

12. Identifying Excuse-making. Look at your action step and identify all of the excuses you make for why you don't carry it out.

13. Understanding Moderation. Complete the food addicts questionnaire (foodaddicts.org/am-i-a-food-addict) and follow the post-assessment instructions. If you've determined that you're not a food addict, make a list of your trigger foods.

14. Practising Mindful Eating. Practise mindful eating by being intentional about what you eat. You will begin by properly plating your meal, moving slowly and relaxed as you prepare to eat. Start by thanking God for the meal and everything that went into getting the food to your table, including the truck drivers, store clerks, field workers, farmers, bakers, etc. Be sure you're sitting at a table instead of standing or eating on the run. Engage all of your senses as you eat. Notice the colours in your food. What does it smell like? Pay attention to the variety of textures. Enjoy all of the different tastes—is it sweet, savoury, salty, or tangy? Then chew your food deliberately and slowly, taking time to put your fork down between bites.

15. Overcoming Excessive Snacking. Challenge yourself to eat only at breakfast, lunch, and dinner—no snacking.

16. Listening to Your Body. With a journal on hand, listen to how your body is talking to you. Pay attention to signals of hunger, gas, bloating, energy levels, overeating, and mood.

17. Overcoming the Spirit of Gluttony. Repent today for your spirit of gluttony. Pour your heart out to God and let Him know your true desire to stop. Write out all the feelings, thoughts, and fears that come up and turn them all over to Him. Then thank Him for hearing and helping you overcome food temptations. Practice watching and praying before you eat anything (Matthew 26:41).

18. Practise Staying Full. Practise praying ceaselessly. Pray as soon as you wake up, giving God thanks for everything you do. Pray as you move from one room to the next and one activity to the next. Pray before

you talk to anyone and pray for anyone that crosses your path. And of course pray before you eat and after you eat.

19. Eating 'Your Food' Only. Make a list of all 'Your Foods' then post it on your fridge or somewhere that you can see it often. Include all the foods you enjoy eating, that taste good, and satisfy you. Make it a point to enjoy those foods today and as often as you can.

20. If you feel like you deserve a treat, pay attention to your entitlement or fairness (or lack of fairness) thinking. Journal them and then use God's Word to confront your beliefs.

21. Food Lies. Write out all the 'lies' you tell yourself when you don't practise your action step that you committed to.

22. Grateful Eating. Pray before all of your meals today, being intentional to change up your routine prayers.

23. Mindful Eating. Pay attention to how often you think about food in unhealthy ways throughout the day. Offer up a prayer, declaration, or confession every time you notice yourself thinking about food at inappropriate times.

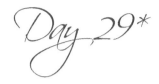

*Day 29**

Fasting for Breakthrough

Scripture Reflection

"Is not this the fast that I choose: to loose the bonds of wickedness, to undo the straps of the yoke, to let the oppressed go free, and to break every yoke?" ~Isaiah 58:6

Devotion

Spiritual Fasting

Fasting is defined as "abstinence from all or some foods or drinks for a set period of time".

It is one of the most powerful weapons God has given us for our daily lives. Through fasting, you can experience spiritual renewal and spiritual breakthroughs in areas you've been bound to. Spiritual fasting is a time of bringing the body under the control of the Holy Spirit on a consistent basis. Although weight loss may result from spiritual fasting, it should not be used in this manner.

Here are the many benefits:

1. It improves your ability to hear from God (Ezra 8:21).
2. It builds you up spiritually (Matthew 4:2, 23, 24).
3. It lifts oppression and breaks demonic powers (Mark 9:29, Isaiah 58:6-8).

4. It leads you into a time of humility and repentance (Psalm 109:22-26).

5. It causes health to spring forth speedily (Isaiah 58:8).

Nutritional Fasting

In addition to the spiritual benefits, fasting has been shown to have many health benefits. It is based on the premise that when you give your body a break from the work of digesting and processing food, it begins to heal itself. It is also based on the premise that when our insulin levels are depleted for long enough, we're able to burn off fat.

Other benefits:

1. It aids in weight loss by boosting metabolism.

2. It reduces insulin resistance.

3. It decreases inflammation in the body.

4. It improves blood and cholesterol levels.

5. It may boost brain function.

6. It could delay aging.

If you want to see all the research studies on the benefits of fasting, see footnote[11].

Types of Nutritional Fasting

INTERMITTENT FASTING.

An eating pattern that cycles between periods of fasting and feeding/eating which could look like no eating from 7pm-7am (12-hour fast), no eating from 7pm-11:00am (16-hour fast) or no eating from 7pm-1pm (18-hours fast). To learn more about intermittent fasting, see footnote[12].

11   https://www.healthline.com/nutrition/fasting-benefits#section4
12   https://www.healthline.com/nutrition/intermittent-fasting-guide

ALTERNATE-DAY FASTING.

On this eating plan you fast every other day, but eat whatever you want on the non-fasting days. You can drink as many calorie-free beverages as you like. Examples include water, unsweetened coffee and tea, and eat about 500 calories on fasting days, or 20–25% of your energy requirements. To learn more about this fast, see footnote[5].

Nutritional fasting is a great tool to implement if you've cleaned up your diet and are exercising consistently, but still don't see much movement on the scale.

I suggest you fast both spiritually to break food strongholds as well as nutritionally to improve your health. Spiritual fasting is very much a Spirit-led journey, whereas nutritional fasting is more of a choice—although it should also be approached after much prayer.

Action

Just for today, you're going to practice the discipline of fasting from 6:00 A.M. to 6:00 P.M. As you fast today, keep a journal and pay attention to what feelings arise. If you're not able to do it, or if you make adjustments, simply journal what adjustments you made and why. (No guilt or condemnation.) Of course, make your necessary adjustments for medications, etc. Always check with your doctor before fasting if you take medication.

Reflect

1. What are you telling yourself about your ability to fast? What fears come up?

In addition to food strongholds, what are some yokes that you believe spiritual fasting can break?

_____

_____

2. How will you either add fasting to your lifestyle or improve your adherence to your current fasting program on a consistent basis?

_____

_____

3. The purposes and benefits of both spiritual and nutritional fasting are essential in your health and weight releasing program. How will you be mindful to make sure that you are not using spiritual fasting to lose weight?

_____

_____

Prayer

"Dear Lord, I thank You that You have provided me with spiritual weapons as well as practical strategies to help me bring my eating under control. I know the benefits of fasting, but I'm so afraid to go without food sometimes. Please lead me into this process of fasting and reassure me that You've got me, that I don't need to be afraid of getting too hungry. I know in my head that You would never command me to fast without giving me the strength to do it, so I am calling out to You today. Tell me how You want me to fast. Tell me what foods You would have me lay down as I feast on Your Word instead. In Jesus' Name, Amen."

Additional Scriptures

"Let not the one who eats despise the one who abstains, and let not the one who abstains pass judgment on the one who eats, for God has welcomed him." ~Romans 14:3 ESV

"And when you fast, do not look gloomy like the hypocrites, for they disfigure their faces that their fasting may be seen by others. Truly, I say to you, they have received their reward. But when you fast, anoint your head and wash your face, that your fasting may not be seen by others but by your Father who is in secret. And your Father who sees in secret will reward you." ~Matthew 6:16-18 ESV

"Why have we fasted, and you see it not? Why have we humbled ourselves, and you take no knowledge of it?' Behold, in the day of your fast you seek your own pleasure, and oppress all your workers. Behold, you fast only to quarrel and to fight and to hit with a wicked fist. Fasting like yours this day will not make your voice to be heard on high. Is such the fast that I choose, a day for a person to humble himself? Is it to bow down his head like a reed, and to spread sackcloth and ashes under him? Will you call this a fast, and a day acceptable to the Lord? "Is not this the fast that I choose: to loose the bonds of wickedness, to undo the straps of the yoke, to let the oppressed go free, and to break every yoke? Is it not to share your bread with the hungry and bring the homeless poor into your house; when you see the naked, to cover him, and not to hide yourself from your own flesh?"
~Isaiah 58:3-7 ESV

* Publisher's note: This day was originally a second 'Day 11' that somehow made it past the author and editors. So rather than just remove it, we've included it here as a bonus for you.

THANK YOU

Thank you for being motivated, courageous, inquisitive, and committed to go deeper into your health journey and uncover the missing piece—Christ!

I pray that these principles have been as much of a blessing to you as they have been for me and the hundreds of thousands of women around the world who have experienced what it means to include God in their health and weight-releasing journey.

If you've been blessed by this book, then please don't keep it a secret!

There are millions of women who need to hear this message. Please take a moment to leave an honest book review so more people can discover this book as well.

This book has laid out a great foundation for you, but there's so much more for you to discover. Please keep in touch with me so that you can stay in this conversation and continue to make your health a priority, God's way. Plus I'll send you a free copy of my *3 Steps to Overcoming Emotional Eating* guide when you enroll for my weekly devotional message on successful weight-loss, God's way.

healthyeatinggodswaybonus.com

Leader's Guide

Healthy Eating, God's Way
Leader's Guide

*"Therefore go and make disciples of all nations,
baptizing them in the name of the Father and of the
Son and of the Holy Spirit, and teaching them to obey
everything I have commanded you. And surely I am
with you always, to the very end of the age."*
(Matt 19:20)

Thank you for answering the call to lead a group through the *Healthy Eating, God's Way* 28-day challenge and devotional. Coming together as a group holds you accountable and provides an opportunity to develop consistency within your faith. The best way to learn is to teach. We believe that as you lead others, you will also continue to grow in the Lord.

Healthy by Design ignites and mobilizes leaders who want to use their spiritual gifts and skills so that others can be transformed by the truth of God's Word.

Know that when you say 'yes' to minister to others, you are changing and affecting not only their lives but also the lives of everyone they come in contact with. You will find that, as a leader, you will feel more connected with the devotionals as you take on a sense of ownership and responsibility and want to support your small group as much as possible.

You have the option of leading the challenge online or in an in-person group. As a leader, you must register your courses with us. Please register your group here:

https://www.cathymorenzie.com/become-a-bible-studyleader/

The 28-day challenge/devotional works best when participants work independently and follow up their independent study with leader-led small-group interaction either in person or virtually.

As the group leader, your responsibility is to facilitate discussion and conversation and make sure that everyone gets the most out of the devotionals. You are not responsible for having all the answers to people's questions or reteaching the content.

That's what the devotional is for.

Your role is to guide the experience, encourage your group to go deeper into God's Word, cultivate an atmosphere of learning and growth amongst a body of believers, and answer any questions that the group may have.

Tips to get the most from the Small Group Sessions

1. It's about God. Although we use biblical principles to guide us on how to address strongholds in our lives, at the end of the day remember that it's always about God. Your role as a leader is to always point everyone to the cross.

2. Partner up. Have your group choose an accountability partner to go through the devotional with. It's always more encouraging when you can connect with someone on a regular basis in addition to when you meet as a group.

3. Keep a journal. Encourage your group to use a supplemental journal. They can choose from an online journal like Penzu (penzu.com) or use old-school pen and paper. Either way, taking time to record your thoughts, feelings, inspirations, and directives from the Holy Spirit is a great way to maximize the experience.

4. Be consistent. Meet at the same time and location each week. This will help the group to organize their time and their schedules. Try to select a time that works best for everyone.

5. Plan ahead. Take time prior to the weekly study to think about how you will present the material. Think about a story or example that would add to the material. Think about the most effective way to make use of the time.

6. Keep it intimate. Keep the small group small. I suggest a maximum of 12-15 people. This will create a more relaxed and transparent atmosphere so that people will feel safe to speak.

7. Be transparent. You can set the tone for the group by sharing your story. This will help people to feel safe and establish trust with them. When you speak, give personal examples and avoid phrases like 'some people' and 'Christians'.

8. Be professional. Always start and end the sessions on time. Communicate clearly if you see that you will be going over-time. Apologize and let them know how much you respect their time.

9. Bring lots of energy. Let your passion for studying God's Word be evident. Remember that your energy level will set the tone for the entire group, so bring it!

10. Pray. It might sound obvious, but make sure that prayer is an intricate part of the entire process. Pray at the beginning and end of every session. Feel free to call on others to lead the prayers. During the session, you can have one person pray for the entire group—have one person open and another close—ask for requests, or select someone. You can also encourage the group to pray for one another. Lastly,

don't forget to pray during the time leading up to the session.

11. Keep it simple. If the sessions get too complicated, people will find reasons not to attend. If you plan to serve snacks, keep it simple and nutritious. Don't plan weekly potlucks that will require the group members to do too much work.

12. Be creative. Feel free to add music, props, or anything that you feel will add to the environment and facilitate learning.

13. Be comfortable. Make sure there is adequate comfortable seating for everyone. Check the temperature in the room. Alert everyone as to where the bathrooms are located.

Preliminary Preparation

- Pray and seek the Holy Spirit on whether you should participate in this devotional.

- Determine with your group how long you will meet each week, so you can plan your time accordingly.

- Most groups like to meet from one to two hours.

- Promote the challenge and devotional through community announcements, social media, in your church bulletin, or simply call a few of your friends.

- Send out an email to a list or send a message on social media announcing the upcoming devotional and challenge.

- Prior to the first meeting, make sure that everyone purchases a copy of the devotional. Include a link where they can buy it.

- Have the group read Day 1 and be prepared to share their responses.

Suggested Group Plan

Because *Healthy Eating, God's Way* is an independent devotional and challenge, the group discussion will incorporate a series of small discussions within the greater discussion. Feel free to customize the design to fit the needs of your group. The suggested plan is for a four-week session. Following is the breakdown.

A Four-Week Session Plan

Session 1

1. Welcome everyone to the session and open with prayer.

2. Share a bit about yourself. Then go around the room and have everyone introduce themselves. Have each person share what their biggest challenge they experience when it comes to healthy eating.

   What are the challenges and stresses they face? Are they consistent or sporadic? Do they eat emotionally, eat late at night or skip meals?

3. Give an overview of the devotional and a brief overview of the *Healthy Eating, God's Way* challenge and devotional. Read the Day 1 Devotional, *Food as a Gift From God* and ask your group if they are ready to commit to the process.

4. Housekeeping Items:
   - format for the session
   - confirm dates and times
   - where bathrooms are
   - rules for sharing
   - commitment to confidentiality

- attendance each week
- snacks (have volunteers provide)

5. Offer suggestions to get the most out of the devotional and challenge.

   Ask the group if they will commit to completing the 'Just for Today' challenge everyday. Consider offering weekly incentives or prizes.

6. Stress the importance of trust and transparency.

7. Instruct the group to complete the six days before the next session. Encourage them to carve out some time each day to complete the devotions and to do their chosen level of activity.

8. Review the Day 1 devotion and ask the group to share their responses.

Suggested Discussion Starters:

- What is your current perception of food?
- Have you truly asked God to search your heart and show you what keeps sabotaging you and why you keep taking matters back into your own hands?
- What stops you from developing a consistent healthy eating routine?
- What negative beliefs do you have about healthy eating that sabotages you?
- What difference would it make in your life if you began to see nutritious food as a gift from God?
- How is the Holy Spirit speaking to you?

9. Have the group read Week 2 for next week's session.

10. Close the session in prayer.

Session 2

1. Welcome the group.
2. Start with an opening prayer.
3. Ask the group what insights/breakthroughs/ testimonials they encountered as a result of what the Holy Spirit has been showing them.

Suggested Discussion Starters (from week 2):

- How will planning improve your chances of success?
- Explain the impact of the 'three brains' on your healthy eating journey.
- What was your experience when you practised fasting for one day?
- What was the outcome when you allowed yourself to feel you feeling instead of feeding them?
- Identify up to three excuses you make that prevent you from eating as healthily as you desire.

4. Make a closing remark or statement to tie in the entire conversation.
5. Have the group read week 3 for next week's session.
6. End with a closing prayer.

Session 3

1. Welcome the group.
2. Start with an opening prayer.
3. Ask the group what insights/breakthroughs/ testimonials they encountered as a result of what the Holy Spirit has been showing them.

Suggested Discussion Starters (from week 3):

- Identify some triggers that cause you to overeat?
- What two or three mindful eating suggestions did you practise and what difference did it make?
- Do you snack out of true hunger or habit?
- As you listened to how your body is always speaking to you, what did you hear?
- When it comes to food and healthful eating, does your public and private life line up?
- Jesus tells the disciples to 'watch and pray.' As it relates to your healthful eating journey, what do you need to watch and pray about most?

4. Have the group read week 4 for next week's session.
5. End with a closing prayer.

Session 4

Think about how you will make the final session memorable. Maybe end with a group walk, do one of my exercise videos together, or give out little rewards to the group's commitment to exercise.

1. Welcome the group.
2. Start with an opening prayer.
3. Ask the group what insights/breakthroughs/ testimonials they encountered as a result of what the Holy Spirit has been showing them.

Suggested Discussion Starters (from week 4):

- What scriptures minister to you most that keep you on track with healthful eating?

- Share a few foods from your healthy eating food list. What foods most energize you?
- What will you do the next time you feel that you deserve a treat or something outside of your boundaries?
- What are some lies you tell yourself about food or eating that lead you to sabotage your efforts?
- Reflect on your mealtime prayers. How can you "spice them up?"
- How do you put yourself in compromising situations that make it difficult to maintain your boundaries? What will you do differently next time?
- How has the Holy Spirit been speaking to you?

4. Wrap up the session with closing words/thoughts. Encourage the group to continue the great work that they've begun.

5. End the session with a closing prayer.

Thank you again for taking the time to lead your group. You are making a difference in the lives of others and having an impact on the Kingdom of God.

Other *Healthy by Design* Offerings

Healthy by Design (healthybydesignprogram.com) equips women to rely on God as their strength so they can live in freedom, joy, and peace. At the end of the day, that's what we really want. Let's be honest, if you never achieved that mythical, elusive number on the scale, but were fully able to live a life of freedom, joy, and peace, would that be enough? I know for me the answer is a resounding 'YES!!!'

We provide a multidimensional approach to releasing weight. It encompasses the whole person—spiritual, psychological, mental, nutritional, physical, and even hormonal! We believe that you must address the whole person—body, soul, and spirit. If you're looking for a program that just tells you what to eat and what exercises to do, this ain't it.

This program has helped thousands of women break free from all the roadblocks that have been hindering their weight loss success while discovering their identity in Christ.

Healthy by Design offers a variety of free and paid courses and programs. They include the following:

The *Weight Loss, God's Way* Devotional Newsletter

Join the free *Weight Loss, God's Way* community and receive regular posts designed to help you align your weight loss with God's Word. You'll also receive a special bonus gift just for joining. To join the newsletter, sign up at:

healthyeatinggodswaybonus.com

Bible Studies for Churches and Small Groups

The membership program can also be experienced a la carte with a group of your friends or with your church. Take one of our three-to-six week studies on a variety of health and weight-releasing topics. To learn more about starting a Bible study in your home or church, go to:

https://www.cathymorenzie.com/start-a-wlgw-group/

Books and Devotionals

You can find all of our *Healthy by Design* series of weight loss books here:

Christianweightlossbooks.com

Keynote Speaking

Want me to visit your hometown? Need a speaker for your annual conference or special event? My fun and practical approach to *Weight Loss, God's Way* will give your group clarity and focus to move toward their weight loss goals. To learn more or to book a speaking engagement, visit:

https://www.cathymorenzie.com/speaking/

Private Coaching

Prefer a more one-on-one approach? I have a few dedicated time slots available to coach you individually to help you fast-track your results. To learn more, go to:

https://www.cathymorenzie.com/coach-with-cathy-2/

Other *Healthy by Design* **books by Cathy Morenzie:**

Weight Loss, God's Way:
The Proven 21-Day Weight Loss Devotional
Bible Study

Weight Loss, God's Way:
Low-Carb Cookbook & 21-Day Meal Plan

Pray Powerfully, Lose Weight:
21 Days of Short Prayers, Declarations,
Scriptures, and Quotes for a Healthy Body,
Spirit, and Soul.

Love God, Lose Weight:
Freedom from emotional eating, overeating,
and self-sabotage by accepting God's Love

Get Active, God's Way:
Weight Loss Devotional and Workout
Challenge

About The Author

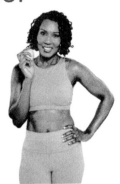

Cathy is a noted personal trainer, author, blogger and presenter, and has been a leader in the faith/fitness industry for over a decade. Her impact has influenced hundreds of thousands of people over the years to help them lose weight and develop positive attitudes about their bodies and fitness.

Over the years, she has seen some of the most powerful and faith-filled people struggle with their health and their weight.

Cathy Morenzie herself—a rational, disciplined, faith-filled personal trainer—struggled with her own weight, emotional eating, self-doubt, and low self-esteem. She tried to change just about everything about herself for much of her life, so she knows what it's like to feel stuck. Every insecurity, challenge, and negative emotion that she experienced has equipped her to help other people who face the same struggles—especially women.

With her *Healthy by Design* books and *Weight Loss, God's Way* programs, Cathy has helped thousands to learn to let go of their mental, emotional, and spiritual bonds that have kept them stuck, and instead rely on their Heavenly Father for true release from their fears, doubts, stress, and anxiety. She also teaches people how to eat a sustainable, nutritious diet, and find the motivation to exercise.

Learn more at www.cathymorenzie.com.

Follow Cathy at:

https://www.facebook.com/weightlossgodsway/

https://www.youtube.com/user/activeimage1

https://www.pinterest.ca/cathymorenzie

Made in the USA
Coppell, TX
19 April 2022

76792424R00103